THE TWO FACES OF RELIGION

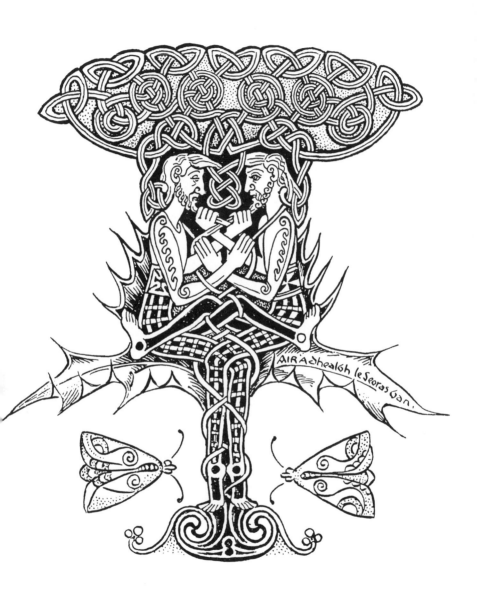

AIR A dhealbh le Seoras Gan

THE TWO FACES OF RELIGION

A Psychiatrist's View

BY

N. S. XAVIER, M.D.

A **PORTALS** BOOK

Portals Press, P.O. Box 1048
Tuscaloosa, Alabama 35403

ISBN 0-916620-86-7

Manufactured in the United States of America

CONTENTS

"Science without religion is lame; religion without science is blind."

— Albert Einstein

"[Religion] has two faces: one the face of truth, the other the face of deception."

— Arthur Schopenhauer

INTRODUCTION

Almost every day—sometimes every hour—of my psychiatric practice I deal with religious/spiritual issues. And I am thoroughly impressed by the tremendous power of religion—both to heal and to harm.

Religion—and its power to help as well as to hurt—is by no means confined to the private world of the individual; it involves families, communities, and nations. Hardly a day goes by without the daily news informing us of tragic consequences from conflicts related to religion. On the other hand, the positive contributions of religion, although less often reported in the news, are truly great.

Clearly, religion has individual and social dimensions, and the two intertwine. Moreover, both of these dimensions have healthy and unhealthy aspects. Understanding the healthy and unhealthy aspects will provide the proper perspective on religion. Selective perception of the negative aspects of religion often leads to rejection of religion; it is like throwing the baby out with the bathwater. However, we can unintentionally become victims of the negative aspects if we are not aware of them. Hence the importance of knowing both sides of religion. The resurgence of religion in recent years—most obviously the rise of fundamentalism in various faiths—makes it particularly relevant and timely for us to examine now the two sides of religion.

Great religious teachers of various times and different cultures have emphasized the importance of following what is truly good in religion, as opposed to the evil disguised as good. Many thinkers in the field of psychiatry also have emphasized the same point and have shown ways to make a distinction between the evil and the good. We will integrate the wisdom of psychiatry and religion for a better understanding of the issue. The Biblical teaching—*judge the tree by its fruits*—makes excellent sense. In fact, the greatest contribution of depth psychology is the understanding of the deeper dynamics of human behavior—far beyond what people consciously profess. The old saying "religion is as religion does" is psychologically quite sound.

The healthy aspects of religion—what enables people to be compassionate, truthful, disciplined, understanding, peace loving, responsible, creative, and open minded—will be referred to as 'healthy spirituality'. At its best it manifests as 'mature spirituality'. The sick side of religion—what makes some religious people hateful, clannish, alienated, fearful, arrogant, destructive, irresponsible, rigid, and closed-minded—will be referred to as 'unhealthy (or sick)

vii

religiosity'. Religious fanaticism is the extreme of sick religiosity. (Fundamentalism and fanaticism are not the same, as will be discussed in Chapter 4.) Only a small percentage of people are at either extreme. The vast majority of individuals involved in religion show varying mixtures of the two aspects. Those who use religion as an occasional social activity or as a forum for business contacts (or to compare clothes, as George Bernard Shaw observed) may show hardly any effects of religion. Like taking inadequate doses of antibiotics, such people may only become resistant to the benefits.

We will examine how the healthy and the sick aspects of religion center around the dynamics of fear, love, and knowledge (including the openness of mind and identity). Therefore in exploring the dichotomy of religion, we will be dealing with many issues that are of great significance both in psychiatry and in religion—the issues of love and hate, ignorance and wisdom, fear and courage, alienation and integration.

The conclusions expressed in this book are derived from the following five sources:

(1) Extensive review of literature.

(2) Discussions and other communications with several hundred individuals active in various religions.

(3) Discussions with nearly two hundred professionals in the fields of psychiatry, social sciences, and the humanities.

(4) My clinical work with patients who are struggling with religious/spiritual issues.

(5) Personal experience.

Although anecdotal examples are given to illustrate certain points, our conclusions are not based on such isolated incidents.

In dealing with the dichotomy in religion, we need to be aware of the danger of 'dichotomous assumption'—assuming that if someone opposes something, he/she is automatically supporting the opposite pole in a dichotomy: for example, assuming that Jane is supporting atheism or communism if she is opposing a Calvinistic ideology. It is as absurd as judging a speech on the problems of obesity to be a speech in support of starvation. While there are real dichotomies in life, it is important to recognize the vast grey areas.

The importance of objectivity is widely recognized in all branches of science. In psychiatry, we are equally impressed by the need for empathy. Special care has been taken here to view the subject matter with objectivity and empathy. At the same time, I do have the clinician's interest in improving health. Our views will reflect a holistic approach rather than a fragmented one.

This is a book on the psychology of religion from a clinician's viewpoint, not a book on comparative religions. Examples and ideas from various religions are used here, not in the spirit of comparing and contrasting different religions as to their intrinsic merits but rather to illustrate and illuminate the psychological factors discussed.

Three decades ago, reviewing the history of religion, Arnold Toynbee observed that it was time to make a fresh start from the spiritual side. He pointed out how the Western World had largely followed the scientific line from the seventeenth century onward. The religious fanaticism of earlier ages—with religious wars, persecutions, and superstitions—had caused many in the West to shy away from religion in the seventeenth century. In calling for renewed spirituality, Toynbee was careful both to warn against the repetition of the extremisms of religion and to advocate the continuation of scientific endeavors.[1]

Religion has faced many struggles since the Middle Ages and has bounced back with varying degrees of renewed strength. Science, while contesting much, did not eliminate religion as some had expected. In fact, many big names in quantum physics—Albert Einstein, Werner Heisenberg, Erwin Schroedinger, and others— were strong believers in spirituality. Secularism in many modern states, while reducing the political clout of religion, is far from eliminating its considerable influence in public life.

Marxism has not succeeded in stamping out religion by the political will of the proletariat. Nor could psychoanalysis analyze away religion as the universal neurosis of humankind. In psychiatry, religion has been gaining more respectability; there is even so-called 'Christian Psychiatry'—a curious cross-breed between Psychiatry and Christian Fundamentalism. And there are 'past-life therapists' who claim to deal with problems arising from traumatic experiences in previous lives. Existentialism has both theistic and atheistic proponents; it has opposed carrying rationalism to irrational extremes.

Psychiatry and religion have many areas of common interest. By working together, both can make immense contributions toward the development of individuals and the progress of societies. This book is intended as a contribution to that worthy cause.

Part One of this book deals with the manifestations of the two faces of religion and the different vantage points from which to view them. A chapter on religious fanaticism and another on mature spirituality are included. The psychological dynamics responsible for the dichotomy in religion (such as fear, courage, narcissism, love/hate, knowledge and identity) are dealt with in Part Two. Part Three gives examples of mature spirituality, religious fanaticism, and clinical examples of spiritual growth. The first chapter of Part I provides the background from which our ideas have developed.

To protect privacy and confidentiality, we have effectively altered the identity of private persons presented herein as examples taken from personal and professional experience.

PART ONE

THE MADNESS AND
THE METHOD

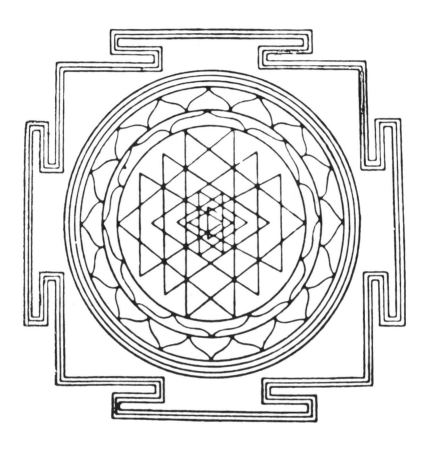

1. HOW THE THEME DEVELOPED

One beautiful but tragic day, John Jr. entered his local church as an apparently quite sane young man. About an hour later, after listening to an intensely emotional sermon, he came out totally insane. In spite of this catastrophe, his family continued to have a strong faith in God; and their faith helped in John's complete recovery some years later.

Both this dramatic real-life incident and the contrasting outcomes of two Hindu converts to Christianity, one doing well and the other going psychotic, were among the happenings I observed during my childhood that made me curious about mental health and its relationship to religion. The seeds of curiosity planted early in life sprouted later and have since blossomed.

In this chapter I will give some examples of the manner in which my interest grew. I will include a clinical example of how ideas expressed in this book helped tremendously in treating one particular case.

A Brief Background: My childhood was spent in the state of Kerala in South India—a state unique in many ways. Sankara, the great Hindu philosopher, was born there. Christianity is believed to have been brought there in the First Century A. D. by St. Thomas the Apostle. My family belongs to the so-called "St. Thomas Christians." During the early centuries of Christianity, Christians and Jews fleeing religious persecution had migrated from the Middle East to Kerala and lived there peacefully. From the Ninth Century A.D., Islam also spread in Kerala. In Kerala various religions— mainly Hinduism, Christianity, and Islam—have existed side by side in peace and harmony on the whole. Even the Hindu-Moslem atrocities of 1947 did not affect Kerala. Nevertheless, fanaticism had existed there on small group and individual levels.

Because various religious groups contributed greatly to the education of its people, Kerala has the highest literacy rate (about 70%) and the lowest population growth rate in India. In fact, international studies on population growth cite Kerala as a good example of population control achieved because of the high literacy rate of women.

My undergraduate and medical school days were spent in Gwalior, about two hundred miles south of Delhi, a stronghold of Hindu fundamentalism. In Gwalior I was exposed to the other religions of India. I became interested in meditation in the sixties when Maharishi Mahesh Yogi made a visit to my medical school. The Maharishi told the assembly of doctors and medical students that the

3

rate of illness can be radically reduced by regular practice of meditation. There was obvious tension in the audience and the speaker sensed the personal concerns of his listeners. He said, "Don't worry about what will happen to your future; you can be the leaders of the healthy." The audience was calm again.

In Gwalior I came to know some victims of communal religious conflict and many individuals ranging from one extreme of religion to the other. Some of these people had risked their own lives to protect members of an opposing community during conflicts. Later, while working in Jamaica, I treated Rastafarians who smoked marijuana as a sacrament and who believed the Emperor Haile Selassie of Ethiopia to be God. Such experiences kept my curiosity about religion alive. Living in the United States for over a decade and being exposed to various religions, spiritual movements, cults, electronic churches, and the like, has deepened my interest and understanding of religion.

Working in the field of psychiatry has given me a special opportunity to understand religious phenomena both conceptually and experientially, through the almost daily experience of treating individuals struggling with spiritual conflicts. After all, psychiatrists are at least supposed to be 'Physicians of the Soul'. Also numerous meaningful coincidences (experiences of 'synchronicity', to use a Jungian term) have helped in developing the ideas expressed in this book. Many people whom I assisted have played a major role in this process.

Examples From Personal Experiences: In my introductory paragraph, I mentioned a case of psychosis precipitated by a religious experience. The details of the young man's case will illustrate the two sides of religion.

In my elementary school days, I knew John Jr. as a rather shy, gentle, hardworking individual. He got along well with his family and neighbors. His father, John Sr., was a well-respected person. He had special skill in treating the various ailments of animals. When domestic animals belonging to his neighbors got sick, John Sr. would treat them without charge. He was a hard-working person and a devout Catholic.

John Jr. was in his mid-twenties when he attended an annual religious retreat in his church. The retreat consisted of three days of lectures, reflections, and prayers. Lectures were given that year by a Franciscan monk. People attending the retreat listened to the lectures; they prayed and some of them also fasted. They took time to reflect on the topics discussed in the talks.

On that particular day of John junior's breakdown, the lecture was on death and on life after death. The monk was an impressive speaker; people liked his style. He stirred up strong feelings in his listeners, especially emotions of fear and guilt. To illustrate his talk, the monk had brought a skull with him. As he spoke, he pointed at the hollow sockets and talked about how the eyes of the dead person could have committed sins by looking at forbidden objects. He pointed out that perceptions from the eyes could have led to evil thoughts and evil deeds. He directed the attention of his listeners to the mouth of the skull and warned them about sins committed by evil speech, lies, and so on.

The monk went on to describe hell-fire and damnation, the terrible pain of Hell, and experiences in Purgatory. He pictured the devils with their pitchforks putting more and more fire on the sinner to keep him/her burning. The lecture lasted about an hour; people listened intensely.

John Jr. was tense, frightened, and shaky. He waited for the last minute of the talk, then got out as fast as he could through the crowd. When he got outside, he knelt on the ground of the churchyard, and started shouting. He was praying and singing and "talking out of his head." He had lost touch with reality. He had been apparently quite sane when he went inside the church that morning. He had no history of psychosis or any emotional problems before that day. He had always been interested in work and family life and had several close friends. No particular stress had been evident in his life. The psychosis was clearly precipitated by the experience at the retreat.

John's mother, however, had suffered from what appeared to be chronic schizophrenia, and he therefore had a genetic predisposition for this condition. His father had only two choices when John Jr. lost touch with reality. He would have to send his son to a state mental hospital quite far from home, or treat him at home. That was before the days when psychiatric facilities became readily available close at home in Kerala.

John Sr. decided to take care of his son at home, where treatment would be with indigenous medicines that he could prepare himself. Since John's mother was suffering from schizophrenia, she could not be of much help. With a tremendous effort, the father did effectively care for his son. Having to help with the personal hygiene and prepare the medication required hours of hard work. At the same time, the father had to carry on his regular responsibilities as a small farmer. In some way, he found the strength to do it all.

John's mental condition was poor; he was in a regressed state. He had to be chained to a heavy block of wood to keep him from running away. He had to be cleaned, fed, and comforted. Those efforts continued day in and day out for several years. There would be some signs of progress, only to be followed by regression. I would consider his diagnosis to be chronic schizophrenia. After about four years, the improvement became more steady. Finally, John Jr. regained full touch with reality; after another few months, he started working again.

Soon he began socializing, going to church, and taking his place as a fully adjusted member of society. His basic gentleness and caring remained, but he became more outgoing than he was before the psychotic episode. I have never again seen such a remarkable recovery in a patient suffering from chronic schizophrenia.

John's recovery was accomplished through the good care that he received from his family, largely from his father, though other family members had also assisted. What enabled the family to bear up through all those months and years when John was in such an unhappy state? What gave them the hope that he would improve and made it possible for them to nurture and sustain him?

Their strong religious faith gave them the hope and the strength they needed. While some people would have become bitter toward the church and the monk who had brought John to his breakdown, the spiritual faith of his family upheld them. They did realize, however, that overemphasis on hellfire and damnation could result in the kind of illness that had afflicted John.

The two conversions I mentioned earlier also deserve careful consideration. Both involve individuals who were converted from Hinduism to Christianity. As a child, I knew both these people, a man and a woman. Let us call the man Matthew and the woman Rosa. The people who encouraged and helped the conversion were also well known to me. Both Matthew and Rosa knew many Christians and, from observing these Christians, they learned about that faith. Matthew's conversion came about rapidly, in a matter of weeks. He was influenced by men who had fanatical tendencies. The women who influenced Rosa to accept Christianity were more on the spiritual side of the spectrum. It is not the intention here to suggest that men are more fanatical in their religious beliefs and women more spiritual but to point out that it was logical for Matthew to be influenced by men and Rosa by women because of the sexual segregation in their society.

Matthew's conversion and subsequent adjustment went fairly well for a few months. He was excited about his new-found faith; his supporters were helpful; and he married a Christian woman. His wife had been born in a Christian family and had grown up as a Christian. Gradually, however, Matthew began having difficulty. He had cut himself off from his relatives, all of whom were Hindus. He became withdrawn, lost interest in the normal activities of daily life and in church attendance.

As Matthew started having problems, his supporters began having doubts about his sincerity in the Christian faith. They suspected that his Hindu relatives were trying to use their personal influence and perhaps some kind of magic or witchcraft to win him back to Hinduism. As Matthew's problems and difficulties grew worse, the support from his Christian friends stopped. Gradually he began to lose touch with reality. Unlike John's dedicated family, Matthew's family was already estranged, and he did not have people who cared enough to go to a lot of trouble to help him. As far as I understand, his wife was afraid, and she returned to live with her parents.

Matthew wandered through the streets. He seemed to enjoy scaring school children. Perhaps because he had worked for my family and had taken care of me, he did not try to scare me. Nonetheless, I was hurt and scared as I saw the change in him.

Out of touch with reality, responding to internal stimuli, making inappropriate remarks, talking out of his head, laughing and giggling inappropriately, Matthew wandered. He ate the free food that people gave him, and after some weeks he just disappeared. This man did not have a family history of mental illness. His mental illness was clearly related to his conversion.

Rosa's case was different. She remained single for several years after she became a Christian. Her Christian friends supported her through times of stress, depression, and doubts. Then she met and married a Christian man, a man who had been brought up as a Christian. Rosa had kept some contacts with her Hindu relatives, and she and her husband seem to be happy in their marriage. Rosa knew Matthew well, and she is pained by what happened to him.

Another case involving religion concerns a man who was nicknamed "Saint James." Saint was apparently a very devout Christian. He attended church regularly, not only on Sundays but every day. He attended special services in nearby churches; he seldom missed any special occasions in any of the churches in the surrounding area. In his own church, he was the loudest and clearest in his prayers. His devotion was impressive.

In his relationship with neighbors, he was considered aloof, but did not cause any big problems. When his wife died early in their marriage, he made several unsuccessful attempts to marry again. His neighbors believed that the attempts to marry again were unsuccessful because of his being a 'religious nut'.

Saint had one major problem—the relationship with his children. He was strict and domineering, a harsh disciplinarian. The children lived in fear of their father. He enjoyed controlling and scaring them. This continued not only when the children were young but when they became adults. He had some peculiar ways of punishing the children that saddened and amazed other people who learned about them. He would beat the children with branches of rose bushes, leaving the thorns intact. He would remove the thorns from one end of a branch so he could hold it without hurting his own hand, and would then beat the children with the other end of the branch. He used to make them kneel for long periods of time and promise that they would never get married.

His children were fortunate in that some spiritually healthy neighbors took a genuine interest in their welfare, showing love and care. These neighbors were able to moderate the father's behavior by talking and pleading with him, and occasionally by threatening him. In fact, when one of the children wanted to marry and the father was threatening them with dire consequences, others had to step in and use counter threats. Finally the marriage took place. Because of the help of those genuinely good neighbors, the children grew up fairly well adjusted.

Another interesting case involved a fierce-looking Hindu who was a part-time healer. He also used to sell palm wine, gamble, and seduce other men's wives. Other Hindus had no respect for him but were afraid of him. Although they talked about him behind his back, when they wanted a demon to be exorcised, they sought his help, and he often gave that help for a reasonable fee. It struck me once that this person's popularity for exorcism was due to his bad character, based on the idea that "it takes a thief to catch a thief." Among Catholics, too, the priests who supposedly specialized in exorcism were considered more or less as evil characters.

Hysterical Conversion Reactions and Possessions: Hysterical phenomena are more common in less developed, less educated parts of the world. Such problems were more frequent when I was growing up. Possessions were seen more often among Hindus, but hysterical conversion reactions were common to all communities, particularly among women of a lower socio-economic class. Conversion reactions used to take various forms—tics, shakes, fainting, seizures and so on. The victims got plenty of attention from family and friends. Stresses were alleviated with the emotional support of everyone and by performing religious rituals.

If therapeutic intervention by one's own religion did not work, some people would turn to another religion. Usually the cure was dramatic and complete, although some people were prone to get similar symptoms under stress later. The element of suggestion is strong in the healing rituals, and the whole atmosphere of the ceremony is conducive to producing a hypnotic state in a sick person. Some rituals obviously give an outlet for guilt and anger. For example, when a nagging mother-in-law crawls on all fours around a temple or church, that act of penitence relieves the woman's guilt and the daughter-in-law's anger.

The term "possession syndrome" denotes the phenomenon of an individual being possessed by god or spirit. It is a worldwide phenomenon with cultural differences in manifestations. It can occur individually or in groups and voluntarily or involuntarily. Voluntary possession by a spirit is claimed to be the power behind some of the traditional healers. Involuntary possession is one way of expressing distress. Many investigators consider it a hysterical phenomenon. Others, psychiatrist Scott Peck for example, believe in demon possession and exorcism. I have not explored these two positions sufficiently to take a stand. The example given below shows the power of suggestion in a particular case.

In this special case described to me by the Catholic priests involved, the victim was a young woman. She and her family were Catholic. She was possessed by the spirit of a relative who had passed away a few months prior to the incident. Being Catholic, the family approached some Catholic priests. The priests did not perform a formal exoricsm. Their other attempts to help the woman had no impact upon her. The family then turned to a Hindu healer, who was known to cure people with such problems. He invited the Catholic priests to witness the ceremony he performed. The healer wore impressive costumes; he chanted and danced around a fire. He beat his drum to the tune of the song and dance. The victim of possession was obviously impressed and appeared to be in a dazed state. When the song and dance reached a crescendo, the healer shouted the demon out of the victim.

The young woman remained in the dazed state for several more minutes and then returned to her usual self. The healer explained to the Catholic priests that the impressiveness of the ceremony had convinced the young lady that her symptoms would disappear. And it worked. He did not try to play one-upmanship with the Catholic priests.

Examples From Professional Experience: Like many young educated people in modern times, I was influenced by the rational "scientific" (the mechanistic model) and behavioral outlook which questioned spirituality—even doubted the existence of the subconscious mind. Hysterical conversion reactions and their removal by treatment impressed upon me, more than anything else, the power of the subconscious mind. It also brought a new interest in hypnosis and psychoanalytic ideas.

My attraction to psychoanalysis was tempered by the fanaticism I encountered in some heavily analytically-oriented psychiatrists. In one instance, a patient who kept begging to try electric shock treatment finally committed suicide because his psychoanalytically-oriented psychiatrist kept turning a deaf ear to the patient's pleas. Such incidents helped to keep my mind open to all schools of psychiatry and beyond. Both the power of suggestion and the neurotic aspects Freudians point out in religion are important to

recognize. But, as we will see in the coming chapters, the healthy and
sick aspects of religion go far beyond such explanations.

In hysterical conversion reactions, psychological conflict is turned
into physical symptom. For example, a young lady whom I saw a few
years ago had paralysis of her left arm, with no physical causes to
account for the dysfunction. Upon interviewing her, it became clear
that the symptom appeared soon after she heard that her steady
boyfriend was going out with another woman. The patient had
suspected something like that, but her boyfriend denied it. His lies
made her furious. She wanted to give the fellow one ringing slap
across his face and say goodbye. That, however, would have been out
of character for her. Under that psychological conflict, the symptom
appeared. Her paralysis was completely cured by suggestion under
hypnosis. Now, can you guess whether she is right-handed or left-
handed? The correct answer is the latter.

Hysterical symptoms are sometimes body metaphors. Lack of
sensation in the top of the head may represent "it blew my top," or
seeing everything in red may represent "I saw red." The most
amusing case of conversion reaction that I have seen was a case of
incontinence in a young lady who worked for a surgeon. She was
having some pain in her back, but her boss did not take the symptoms
seriously nor pay even half the attention to her that he was lavishing
on his patients. This lady was single and was attracted to her boss
who was married, but not too happily.

Evidently the situation was too tempting for the young woman.
The situation continued for a few weeks, and then she developed
urinary incontinence. That alarmed her boss, and she was admitted
to the hospital. Then she got plenty of attention from her employer
and from others. Since no physical cause was found for the
symptoms, I was consulted. In treating her, I found that her
incontinence represented her being "pissed off" at her boss. With
psychiatric help, the symptoms cleared and she developed insight
into her conflict.

The most impressive case of conversion reaction I have treated was
that of a middle-aged black man who was brought to the hospital
emergency room one morning by his family. He was unable to move,
he was mute, and it was impossible to tell whether he could hear. I
was a psychiatry resident at the time. The emergency room physician
and the neurology resident could find no physical cause for his
symptoms, so I was called in. You can imagine how elaborate and
beautiful a psychiatric interview I could conduct. I decided to do a
sodium amytal interview (popularly called "truth serum" test).
During the interview the man reported that the previous night he was
walking home when somebody threatened him with a pistol, stole his

billfold, and pushed him to the roadside. He fell but did not get hurt. He managed to get up and walk home. His home was only a few blocks from the place where he was robbed. Everybody at home was already asleep and he did not wake them. He went to sleep. When he was not up and about as usual the next morning, his family tried to wake him. They realized he could not talk or move and was also incontinent.

His family brought him to the hospital without having any idea of what had happened to him. During the amytal interview, all his symptoms were completely relieved. This dramatic recovery was impressive to the patient and his family, as well as to other physicians. The emergency room physician had been insensitive to psychiatric aspects of medicine up to that time, but was converted to the belief that the mind indeed matters. He had previously asked a psychotically depressed lady (who had a delusion that she was dead) why she came there rather than go to the morgue.

Patients struggling with religious/spiritual issues have been a challenge to me in my psychiatric practice. Besides psychiatric approaches, my personal interest in religious and philosophical ideas became useful in dealing with spiritual issues. In this process, my interest in the field deepened, and I tried to understand the healthy and unhealthy aspects of religion. The phenomena of cults and rising fundamentalism, as well as spiritual movements in various parts of the world, further challenged my research. Many of the observations and conclusions expressed in the coming chapters were used clinically to help people. One such case is given below.

Liz is a genuinely caring person who is always willing to extend a helping hand to others if she can. That quality has made her vulnerable to manipulation by some people from time to time. She is deeply loving, open-minded, prudent, and fairly courageous.

The religious fanatic involved in this case is Elaine, who had been a psychotherapist for many years. She became more involved with religion as she grew older. When the company she was working for required her to do more administrative work, she found herself under excessive stress. The company had become more profit-oriented, too, so Elaine was fired from her job. Dr. Brown, a friend, and his nurse Liz, felt sad about Elaine's situation because of her age, her lack of family support, and her loss of a job. These friends helped her set up her own practice. Dr. Brown provided her an office free of charge. Elaine came to know Liz and Dr. Brown more closely. She appeared to be appreciative of their efforts to help and of their compassion. The three of them discussed religious issues many times because all three were interested in that subject. Elaine had strong

Christian fundamentalistic ideas and affiliations, stronger than the other two realized. She would fit Rev. Jerry Falwell's description of "hyper fundamentalist" (see Chapter Four). Later on it became clear that she was-fuming inside when she listened to Dr. Brown's ecumenical christian ideas which Liz shared. Elaine did not show her bad feelings directly, nor did she offer to pray for Dr. Brown and Liz to see light. She did go on to attack them subtly. Her best opportunity for that came when Liz was hospitalized for a surgery. She told Liz that her illness was God's chastisement for her religious belief (that differed from Elaine's) and because of her working for Dr. Brown. Moreover, Elaine warned Liz that the next step for Liz would be death and damnation. According to Elaine, all the inhumane things she was doing were done at the direction of Jesus. Although she was formally affiliated with a traditional Christian church, in reality she was more active in ministries of healing and demon deliverance. She had been casting out demons (demons of lust, sickness, etc.) from gullible people.

Liz was distressed but could not reveal to Dr. Brown what Elaine was doing for fear that it might hurt him. The repeated preaching and threats made by Elaine began to make Liz increasingly nervous and upset after discharge from hospital. She became depressed and her 'nervous stomach' got worse. Soon she experienced severe anxiety and began to think that Elaine and her fanatical church people might be right. She was deeply hurt about the underhanded way Elaine was attacking her and Dr. Brown; but, at the same time, she felt that Elaine might be right in doing so. Elaine could see that Liz was getting worse, but instead of letting up, she pushed Liz all the more. Finally, Liz confided in a friend about Elaine's actions. That friend went to Dr. Brown and informed him what had been happening.

He was pained and shocked by Elaine's evil work done in the name of Jesus. He referred Liz to me for treatment.

When I discussed the situation with Liz, it became clear that Elaine had opened up an old wound of Liz's. Liz had several traumatic experiences with religion as a child and teenager. Her family belonged to the Church of God and Liz was raised very strictly. Movies, dancing, ball games, and even cutting hair were considered sinful. The church used scare tactics by telling her that God would strike her dead for deviating from the Church's ways. As Liz grew up, she noticed the hypocrisy and hatred that were evident in the lives of her church people. Being a loving and honest person, she had serious doubts about their claims. She began searching for a more genuinely spiritual church.

When she was in the process of the search, leaders in the Church of God tried hard to control her by using scare tactics. They sent threatening letters, even skeletons with chains. That did scare Liz; in fact, it caused her severe anxiety for a while.

She did not give up her search for truth, however, nor did she turn her back on her love and goodness. She finally decided to become an Episcopalian. She was not a fanatic Episcopalian either; she chose the healthy side of the religious spectrum. In the meantime, the minister of the Church of God in which Liz had previously been a member was sentenced for sodomy involving a fourteen-year-old boy and had been put in jail. Apparently he had abused many boys sexually.

The frightening experiences Liz had with the Church of God left their mark on her mind. Similar situations used to make her uneasy but not panicky for any length of time. However, when Elaine opened the old wounds, Liz began to suffer from severe anxiety and palpitations off and on for several weeks. Anti-anxiety medications helped her to some extent. What proved most helpful was our discussion of the spiritual issues involved and the psychology of healthy spirituality and unhealthy religiosity, as expressed in this book. She read and re-read the early draft of the chapters on Mature Spirituality and Religious Fanaticism. That helped greatly in clarifying her confusion and in putting matters in the right perspective. At the time when anxiety and palpitations were severe, hypnosis was also used with good results.

Liz had the dynamic of healthy spirituality already but it was not too strong. Her understanding of religion was not quite clear and deep. With Elaine's attack, the old fears, guilt, and confusion from childhood resurfaced. Liz's husband and family were on the fanatical side of religion, and were not helpful. She consulted two priests (the second when the first was away) during the three months of intense struggle. The first one helped her and reinforced her sound ideas about spirituality. The other priest was helpful at times, but at other times his counsel was harmful for he would arouse in her the same kinds of fears and doubts that Elaine had caused. Liz was strong enough to recognize that this latter priest was not a well-integrated person himself, and she quit consulting him.

When Liz improved, she started working for Dr. Brown but continued her therapy. Elaine moved out of Dr. Brown's office but reportedly continued in her fanatical faith. For Elaine, the qualities of love, wisdom, and courage had no real significance, although she paid lip service to them when it suited her. Dogmatic belief in a narrow Christian faith was all that mattered to her. Liz gained clear insight into healthy and unhealthy aspects of religion.

It is my hope that the examples given so far have revealed the background from which my concerns and ideas have developed.

2. FROM CHAOS TO ORDER

"To the corruptions of Christianity I am, indeed, opposed; but not to the genuine precepts of Jesus himself."

— Thomas Jefferson

"Nothing has made more for peace and love than religion; nothing has engendered fiercer hatred than religion."

— Swami Vivekananda

Religion is not just complex; it is quite confusing in many ways. The most paradoxical or contradictory aspect of religion is its strong tendency and tremendous power to do good as well as evil. This is not just a periodic phenomenon, but a consistent aspect of history. In this chapter we will first examine the confusing picture of religion and then try to clarify the confusion.

I. The Confusing Scenario of Religion. Let us take the example of the Golden Rule—"Do unto others as you would have them do unto you." All the great religions of the world subscribe to this principle, although they have expressed it in slightly different ways. And there are plenty of practitioners of these faiths who genuinely try to follow the golden rule—but there are many others who do not try. The end result is that *while the golden rule glitters like gold in the beauty of its principle, it is often as dead as a piece of metal in its practice.* Reflecting the paranoia of our age, Rabbi Abraham Heschel remarked that the modern version of the golden rule is: *"Suspect thy neighbor as thyself."* George Bernard Shaw's version of the golden rule is worth remembering, too: We must *not* do to others as we want them to do to us because their taste may be different from ours.

Let us look at some specific examples of good principles being overlooked or contradicted in various religions. Take Jesus' Sermon on the Mount (the Beatitudes). Many Christians consider it the highest Christian ideal or the maximum Christian virtue. Many other Christians, while paying lip service to it, really live as if the beatitudes were all pure hype (hyperbole)—too good to be true for

14

this world. According to the Beatitudes, the meek and the merciful, the peacemakers, the poor in spirit and those who pursue righteousness are blessed. But if we look at the history of Christianity, frequently the beneficiaries of the Beatitudes were not blessed, but blessed out (cursed).

Look at other religions. The Hindu idea of karma or appropriate consequence to one's actions is an obviously fair principle. But the practice of ill-treating the lower castes shows a lack of concern for karmic consequences. The spirit of social reform and religious toleration of Prophet Mohammed was blocked or reversed by Moslems many times. Fanatic Jews take exception to the Ten Commandments in dealing with Palestinians. Jainism emphasizes non-violence. But many Jains who avoided farming to prevent killing insects reportedly became merchants and money lenders who exploited fellow human beings. Sikhism, which originated as a religion of harmony and peace, has become a source of tragic conflicts in recent years at the hands of extremists. A Sikh gentleman summarized the religious problem thus: "Hindus think and don't act; Moslems act and then think; Sikhs act and never think."

Religious followers also show a strong tendency to revert to the old ways opposed by their founder. Many Buddhists went back to the kind of asceticism, pietism, and pettifoggery that the Buddha had discarded. Many Christians reverted to the dogmatism, legalism, and exclusiveness that Jesus had staunchly opposed.

It is also not uncommon for the extremists of any religion to commit acts of brutality on their brethren who try to follow the true spirit of their religion. For example, Mahatma Gandhi was assassinated by a Hindu fanatic. In another instance, a 76-year-old Sufi (Islamic mystic)—Mahmoud Mohammed Taha—was publicly hanged in Sudan in 1985 for upholding the spirit of justice and equality in Islam rather than the literal application of its ancient laws. Thousands of Islamic fanatics cheered at the brutal sight of his death. Subsequently he has been honored as a martyr by many other Moslems.

Clinical Examples: Many of my patients who suffer from pessimistic, negative thinking have reported benefits from watching Rev. Robert Schuller's television program because of his positive thinking approach. Several others have reported that Rev. Jimmy Swaggart's preachings cause excessive fear and hate because of his extremely negative attitude towards people with a different world view. (On the other hand, his style draws an enthusiastic response from many in his audience.)

Meditation has become popular and is accepted in medicine as an effective tool to cope with stress. It is also one way Eastern religious influence has spread to the West. Meditation has always been very much a part of Christian monasticism and mysticism, but not so much a part of popular Christianity. In recent years, there has been increasing acceptance of meditation among Christians. But there is another side, a sad one at that, to the same story. There are Christians who abhor meditation, especially if it has even a remote connection to Eastern religion. For them it is all a work of the devil. In fact, these Christians view meditation as evidence of the subtlety and the cleverness of the devil seeking to catch innocent people in the net of vices.

I dealt with a clinical case involving this problem —the case of Jill, a young Christian woman. She had functioned fairly well and used meditation to cope with her stresses. She had learned meditation from somebody who was taught by a yoga teacher. She had previously lived in a cosmopolitan city in the northern part of the United States.

After moving down South, she found herself in a neighborhood surrounded by fanatic Christians. Jill is a rather suggestible person with a strong need for acceptance and approval. Moving to a new place and having to take care of her two-year-old boy without help from any reliable relatives put her under considerable stress. Also, her husband was away from home more and their relationship was unhappy. The new friends were unpleasantly surprised that a good Christian girl was meditating. Now they knew why she was stressed and unhappy. The devil had gotten into her. They told her that she would be happy once she got rid of the demon of meditation, thereby improving her personal relationship with Jesus Christ. Jill went along and did as the friends told her, but she had conflicts about it. Because of multiple stresses in her life at the time, Jill gradually developed a clinical depression. With treatment, Jill gradually overcame her depression and also realized how useful meditation had been for her in handling stress. Many of her confusions about what is healthy in religion were clarified.

Fundamentalists of all religions pay great attention to women's clothes. With Islamic revival in many parts of the world, the totally oppressive 'purdah' is more prevalent again. Similarly, some Christian fanatics are terribly opposed to women wearing pants. An interesting case involved a young woman who has always worn pants and doesn't like to wear dresses. She is really modest and nobody had criticized her wearing pants until a few months ago when she had joined a new church along with her whole family. The minister of this new church was a fanatic, particularly harsh with women. Sunday after Sunday he preached against women wearing pants, among other things that would lead to eternal damnation. Our young woman got scared. Her mind was in a way torn beween pants and heaven. She finally decided to wear pants and go back to her old church "whatever the hell might happen." And she did well.

On one occasion I asked a minister who was preaching against women wearing pants what was the basis for his objection. He argued that men and women should wear different kinds of clothes to keep the God-given differences of gender. Since I looked unconvinced he added a last and final statement, "it is all clearly said in the Bible; we either follow the Word of God or be damned forever."

Compassion Versus Exploitation: Charity and compassion are essential virtues in all religions; some groups emphasize it more than others. Various religious groups are providing shelters for the homeless, food for the starving, education for the poor, care for the sick, and counseling for the troubled all over the world.

Mother Teresa is an outstanding example of the millions of people who are devoted to the service of others because of their spiritual ideals. While some Christians have been almost rejoicing about AIDS (Acquired Immune Deficiency Syndrome) as a just punishment from God, Mother Teresa has been trying to help the victims of this fatal disease.

The numerous examples of people who show altruism and sublimation because of their religious ideals raise another important point. Psychiatry teaches altruism, sublimation, and humor as mature psychological defenses. (See psychological defenses in Appendix.) However, one doesn't hear of any outstanding examples of altruism and sublimation coming out of the inspiration of these psychiatric theories. It may be that the news pays less attention to good news. There is something to President Reagan's complaint one time about the "Evening Blues" (evening news). However, I suspect that it is not the news that is at fault in this matter, but that psychiatry does not have the power of inspiration that religion has. Isn't it said that he who can does, and he who cannot teaches? On the flipside of that coin, it is equally true that psychiatry does not do the kind of harm religion does.

While the good side of religion is charitable, the evil side of religion is exploitative. Religion has directly and indirectly exploited vast numbers of people; in fact, religion may be the most effective tool of exploitation that humankind has ever used. Exploitation of women and minorities, slavery, and colonialism were all supported and sanctified in many ways by different religious groups at different times. It is also true that religion has played a significant role in bringing about social justice. Mahatma Gandhi and Martin Luther King, Jr. are good examples. Similar to the issue of compassion versus exploitation is the issue of violence and nonviolence in religion.

Violence and Non-violence: Religious conflicts are one of the major roots of many, if not most, wars and aggressions going on all over the world. Christians and Moslems fight in Lebanon; two different sects of Moslems fight in the Iran-Iraq war; and Arabs and Israelis have been at each other for several decades now. Moslems and Catholics fight in the Philippines; Protestants and Catholics in Northern Ireland; Hindus and Moslems as well as Sikhs and Hindus in India; Buddhists and Hindus in Sri Lanka, and so on. These are the tip of the iceberg with so many more conflicts going on at the local, interfamily, and interpersonal levels

We see members of various religions actively involved in peace movements. We also see other members of the same religions involved in supporting militarism. The nuclear issue is a good example. Religion is a strong opponent of the nuclear arms race in one way. The Methodist Bishops strongly oppose nuclear arms. When the American Catholic Bishops published a pastoral letter opposing an arms race, particularly the nuclear one, and proposing several steps for bringing about international peace, it was supported by some religious groups and opposed by others. Some Christian (including Catholic) *think tanks* tried to shoot down the ideas. Some even argued that Bishops had no business to talk about a military issue, disregarding the fact that this is the ultimate life-and-death issue humankind has faced.

In June, 1982, when Billy Graham attended an international conference on nuclear issues in the Soviet Union, it stirred up political and religious controversy in the United States. Some Christian groups want America to build more nuclear weapons. Also, some of them believe a nuclear holocaust is the way the long awaited end of the world will happen.

What puts the icing on the cake of religion and nuclear armament is the reported plans of Pakistan to produce "Islamic nuclear weapons." As they see it, there are Christian, Jewish, Hindu, Marxist, and Maoist, if not Taoist, nuclear weapons. How spiritually elevating! Doesn't it really sound like finally religion is up to meeting the challenges of the nuclear age? And why not when God's beautiful creations on earth are on the brink of total destruction by *His favorite creatures?* Are we behaving like spoiled children?

While the nuclear threat looms large in the future horizon, political assassination attempts have been among the highlights of the recent past. In September 1981, President Anwar Al Sadat of Egypt, himself a devout Moslem, was assassinated by Islamic fanatics who hated him for signing a peace accord with Israel.

In October 1984, Margaret Thatcher, Prime Minister of England, narrowly escaped an assassination attempted by the IRA (Irish Republican Army). In the same month Sikh extremists assassinated

Indira Gandhi, the Prime Minister of India. Mrs. Gandhi's assassins were two of her own bodyguards, *symoblizing how religious fanaticism destroys the ones it is supposed to protect and nurture.* The English word 'assassin' itself has a religious origin. It is derived from the Arabic word 'hashishiyin' meaning hashish smokers. The 'hashishiyin' were a fanatic sect of Moslems in the middle ages (eleventh to thirteenth centuries). They had a stronghold in Iran, whence their activities spread to the neighboring countries also. Those extremist Shiites believed it their religious duty to kill others whom they considered to be the enemies of true Islam. They infiltrated many communities, charming women with presents of dress and attracting children by giving toys. They treacherously murdered the men whom they wanted to get rid of. Their habit of smoking hashish had earned them the nickname 'hashish smokers'. The Mongols finally crushed their political power. Incidentally, the word 'thug' also has a religious origin. It comes from 'sthaga' (meaning 'cheat' in Sanskrit), a gang of worshippers of Hindu Goddess Kali, who often murdered and plundered.

Two Historical Examples: After the Roman emperor Constantine made Christianity the state religion, power politics became a complicating and often corrupting force in Christianity. One of the interesting and amusing examples of papal abuse of power is the story of Emperor Frederick II of Germany in the 13th century. Pope Innocent III—who showed no innocence in power politics—had supported the selection of Frederick II as emperor. They had an understanding that the emperor would undertake the Sixth Crusade, but he dilly-dallied over making the move. Pope Gregory IX excommunicated the emperor and invaded the German dominons in Italy. Frederick II went to the Holy Land, met with the Sultan of Egypt, reached an agreement, and got part of the kingdom of Jerusalem. Then he returned to Italy, expelled papal armies from his dominions, and pressured the Pope into canceling his excommunication. With these incidents, crusades and excommunications reached the point of *reductio ad absurdum,* as historian H. G. Wells observed.[1]

The next example will show the better side of religion. It is the story of Emperor Asoka, whom H. G. Wells called the greatest of kings. In the Third Century B. C., Asoka ruled a vast empire in Asia which spread from Afghanistan to parts of South India. In the early part of his rule, Asoka invaded a neighboring country successfully. By the standards of traditional political wisdom, one would have expected Asoka to have 'stayed the course' and consolidated his power over the remaining tip of the Indian subcontinent. Even by the tenets of behavioral psychology, one would expect Asoka's expansionist spirits to have been reinforced. But that was not what happened.

The success of his military operations did not go to Asoka's head. Instead, the cruelties and horrors of the war and the immense suffering of the victims touched his heart. Asoka embraced Buddhist teachings, renounced war, and devoted the rest of his life to compassionate work. He became the only military monarch in history who discarded warfare after victory. Asoka organized the digging of wells for drinking water, planting of trees for shade, and the cultivation of herbs for medicine. He founded hospitals for people and for animals. Education was spread throughout his land and special provisions were made for the education of women. Asoka's edicts throughout his land declared the principles of love and peace, and he sent Buddhist teachers to other countries to spread the same message. So impressive was Asoka's rule that H.G.Wells states, in *The Outline Of History:* "Amidst the tens of thousands of monarchs that crowd the columns of history . . . the name of Asoka shines, and shines almost alone, a star."[2] What made Asoka the shining star of history is the light of his genuine and deep spirituality.

Importance of Clarifying the Confusion: The kind of confusion that we have noted has made many people weary of religion. Many have been turned off by the evil side of religion. Many others deal with it only superficially. Many of my colleagues in the mental health profession seem to accept religion as a social phenomenon and not much more. And there are people who think it is a small dose of religion that causes much trouble, that a stronger dose would help the person much more. Indeed, Henry David Thoreau had observed: "We have just enough religion to make us hate, but not enough to make us love one another." Will a stronger dose of religion fix people up? The answer is that it depends on whether we are talking about the healthy or the unhealthy aspects of religion.

When the religious elements are such a mixed bag, it is important to distinguish the good from the bad. We do not give up eating mushrooms just because some varieties of them are poisonous. Similarly, would people give up eating tomatoes because its cousin, nightshade, is poisonous? The akee, an invitingly beautiful fruit found in Jamaica, provides an even more meaningful analogy. Akee is edible when ripe but poisonous otherwise. Something that is potentially nurturing may be actually quite poisonous if consumed unripe and unprocessed. As historian George Marsden said in *Fundamentalism and American Culture,* it is crucial that we distinguish between the true forces for good and the evil powers disguised as angels of light.

II. A Method in the Madness. One may see religion as the ultimate 'good apple with a rotten heart'. Voltaire reportedly thought that religion started at the meeting between the first fool and the first rogue. Some people view religion as a form of politics. In fact, Napoleon had classified the old and new Testaments of the Bible and the Koran under 'politics' in his private library. Nietzsche considered alcohol and Christianity as the narcotics of Europeans. For Marx religion was the opiate of the public, a cause of alienation and a tool of exploitation. As against such cynical attitudes, one can look at religion with a sense of humor and at the commonly used categories of conservative versus liberal, right versus left, from a psychological point of view.

Take It With a Sense of Humor: According to Havelock Ellis, laughter is a religious exercise because it is an expression of the soul's emancipation. At any rate, humor is healthy psychologically and spiritually. The great men and women of religion have shown a fine sense of humor. Guru Nanak, the founder of Sikhism, respected Hinduism and Islam and took good ideas from both. But he also laughed at the many ridiculous practices of both religions. On one occasion he threw water towards the earth saying he was watering his fields in faraway Punjab, when Hindus were throwing water towards the sun as an offering to their ancestors in heaven. On another occasion a Moslem priest was outraged that Nanak was sleeping with his feet toward Mecca. Nanak welcomed the Mullah to turn his feet in any direction where God does not dwell.

Chaucer exposed the superficiality, hypocrisy, narcissism, and greed of a group of pilgrims in "The Prologue" of the Canterbury Tales. He also portrayed a genuinely spiritual parish priest. Among the group was a nun, a prioress who spoke in French. She fed her dogs rich food while a great many people were starving. A "fat and personable" monk enjoyed hunting and giving presents to pretty girls and making money, even sweet talking a poor widow into giving him her little savings. The physician member of the team had specialized knowledge in his profession but cared little for the Bible; he showed off his wealth, although tight with money. The bottom line about the physician, literally and figuratively, was that he loved gold. A Pardoner, licensed by the church to sell pardons, made a fortune out of selling pig's bone (supposedly holy relics) to unsuspecting believers. But the parish priest was sincere, dedicated, humble, and loving. He set a good example.

Mark Twain had a field day of fun, in his *Letters From the Earth,* with some of mankind's most sacred beliefs and their inconsistencies. Human beings who enjoy sexual intercourse more than anything else on earth would replace sex with prayer in Heaven. In Heaven, everybody will be singing all the time, although man cannot stand anything remotely resembling that on earth. As against all the distinctions and discriminations of color and class on earth, in Heaven all are brethren. In the life here Man cares so much about his intelligence, but he couldn't care less about it in the hereafter. Twain found the ideas of creation amusing. It took millions of years of preparation for the coming of man. Fish cultures and formation of coal (for frying fish) and creation of reptiles were part of the process. Man is the cruel and unreasonable animal and the only patriot. "He is the only animal that has the True Religion—several of them. He is the only animal that loves his neighbor as himself, and cuts his throat if his theology isn't straight."[3]

Conservative Versus Liberal Outlook: There are healthy and unhealthy aspects to both conservatism and liberalism. Ultimately what is important is whether it is the healthy aspect one is referring to or the unhealthy one. Spiritually mature individuals possess healthy aspects of both conservatism and liberalism and show very little of the negative elements of either.

The strong points of conservatism include caution, self-control, strong commitment to whatever one identifies with, law and order, consistency and dependability, sense of duty, and a strong sense of right and wrong. Some features such as goal orientation and rationalism can be healthy in moderation but unhealthy in excess. The weak points of conservatism are rigidity, closed-mindedness, diminished capacity for love and empathy (especially toward anything different), narrow identity, excessive fear, more of a 'having' than a 'being' orientation, and more of 'product' than a 'process' orientation. Dichotomous thinking, excessive tradition, too much importance given to appearance (appearing proper, tough, and good) are other problems. Richard Nixon, former United States President, had once advised Republican candidates to be "conservatives with a heart." He thereby pointed at the heart of the conservative problem—too much head and too little heart.

If the head rules the conservative, the heart runs away with the head of the liberal. The liberal's problems are too much feeling, lack of order and control, tendency to make changes easily, lack of prudence, weak commitment, fussy ideas, and undependability. Liberals are driven by love rather than by fear. But their sweet river of love may not reach anywhere for the lack of adequate river banks to channel the flow. It may all just spill over and get lost.

The healthy side of liberalism is open-mindedness, deep love and empathy, tendency to follow the spirit rather than the letter of the laws and rituals, broad identity, and courage to make changes. In their orientation, 'being' is more important than having; and 'process', more than product.

If we take the example of a spiritually mature person like Thomas Merton, the Catholic monk, was he a conservative or a liberal? One can argue the case on either side. Who could be more conservative than a monk in the twentieth century? However, he spent a great part of his life learning about other religions, psychology, anthropology, and various sociopolitical issues. He was opposed to American involvement in the Vietman war and the arms race. So he was a liberal, too. The truth is that the conservative-liberal classification is inadequate and often misleading. Closely allied to these labels are the right versus left classification, which is also fairly commonly used (or rather misused).

Right Wing Versus Left Wing: The right wing is supposedly conservative and the left wing liberal. There is also the term 'centrist' to accommodate the odd ones. When my dictionary and encyclopedia did not shed light on right/left issues, I decided to waste no more time on trivia. But that was not to be so. In the dark night of my ignorance, I came across a speech by Reverend Sun Myung Moon, founder of the Unification Church, and it enlightened me like a full moon at midnight! According to Reverend Moon, the struggle between the right and the left started at Calvary when Jesus was crucified along with two thieves. The thief who was crucified on Jesus' right side accepted and respected Jesus, whereas the thief on the left side rejected him. At that time, the seed for the God-denying world, the present day communist world, was sown by the thief on Jesus' left-hand side. And the seed for the God-fearing world, the free world, was sown by the thief on Jesus' right-hand side. America is the center of the God-fearing world and the defender of God.

Like the experience of Alice in Wonderland, the right/left issue becomes more and more curious if we consider the findings of Roger Sperry and others about the functions of the right and left cerebral hemispheres and the Spiegels' findings on hypnotizability. The left hemisphere mode is characterized by dominance of verbal, mathematical, and analytical processes. These also correlate with low hypnotizability.[4] So the leftists in terms of cerebral lateralization are the conservatives and leftists are less suggestible. What has been said so far has shown the inadequacy of conservative-versus-liberal or right-versus-left classifications. What is more important is to classify the healthy versus the unhealthy aspects of religion.

A Psychological View of Religion: William James noted the following characteristics in healthy-minded religion: joyousness, freedom, optimism, liberal theology, pluralistic views, and absence of preoccupation with sin. On the other hand the 'sick soul' manifests the opposite qualities: melancholy, pessimism, orthodox theology, and preoccupation with sin. Sigmund Freud focused on the negative aspects of religion and interpreted religion as an illusion to fulfill our wishes for protection and immortality. He considered mystical experience as an 'oceanic' feeling—a grandiose compensation for the sense of helplessness. Carl Gustav Jung found the myths and symbols in religions highly beneficial in healing the splits in our psyche. He also noted that spiritual quest makes people's lives meaningful. While he had mixed feelings about organized religion, he strongly supported personal spirituality and built bridges to Eastern thinking.

In *Psychoanalysis and Religion* Erich Fromm dealt with the dichotomy of religion between authoritarian and humanistic polarities. Abraham Maslow observed in *Religions, Values and Peak Experiences* that religion can be divided into left wing (those who have peak experience, or "peakers") and right wing ("non-peakers"). Gordon Allport (in *The Individual and His Religion*) wrote about mature and immature religious sentiments.

The attempt in this book is to view the dichotomy of religion from a broad perspective. For that purpose, we will utilize many areas of knowledge in the wide spectrum of psychiatry and behavioral sciences. Such areas of knowledge include the psychology of group dynamics; identity issues, deeper understanding about fear, love, hate, selfishness, moral reasoning; and the psychology of self-deception. Moreover the wisdom arising from the dialogue between the spiritual traditions of the East and the West will also be used to enrich our overall understanding of the dichotomy in religion.

As mentioned in the introduction, the processes of unhealthy religiosity and healthy spirituality are the opposite forces in the dynamics of religion. The dynamic factors involved in these two processes are centered around fear and love as two basic human motivations. Not only many great thinkers of modern times but also political figures like Nicolo Machiavelli and Napoleon Bonaparte recognized these two motivational factors. These are factors we share with the animal kingdom, although we are much more capable of both love and fear. Another basic motivating factor is centered around knowledge. To know or not to know is a big question for us human beings—perhaps the biggest question, and the one in which we are furthest removed from all the rest of the animal kingdom. So we will try to understand religion, both sides of it, based on these motivational or dynamic factors. Our sense of identity is an integral part of our self-knowledge, and therefore how identity and religion interact will be given due consideration.

Unhealthy religiosity involves excessive fear or lack of prudence, selfishness or self-hate, and hate of others, as well as ignorance and closed-mindedness. These factors lead to conflicts and result in stunted emotional and spiritual growth or destructiveness. Each of these factors will be discussed in detail in the following chapters.

Healthy spirituality involves love of oneself and others, courage and prudence as well as knowledge and open-mindedness. These factors work together to make a person well integrated. True knowledge and open-mindedness constitute wisdom. High integration and wisdom go hand in hand.

According to St. Thomas Aquinas, the cardinal virtues are: wisdom, temperance, courage, and justice. Temperance is caution. And justice is part of love, as we will see in the discussion on love, however, love is a much more basic human dynamic. So we can conceptualize mature spirituality with the threefold focus of love, wisdom, and courage/prudence. This point of view is also consistent with the traditional wisdom of the East and the West regarding the three aspects of the function of our psyche: mind, emotion, and will.

Aristotle observed that virtue is the golden mean and vices are the extremes on both sides of the mean. His idea can be applied to both fear and love:

Vice	Virtue	Vice
Hate of Self/Others	Love of Self/Others	Narcissism, Egoism
Foolhardiness	Courage & Caution	Excessive Fear

However, Aristotle's formula does not work well in the case of knowledge. After all, half truth is not a virtue.

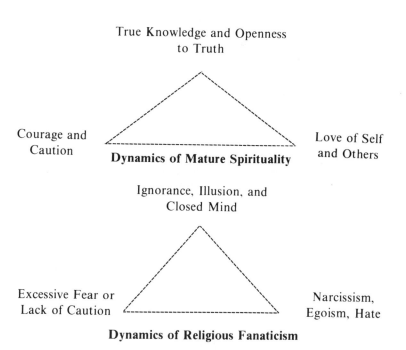

True Knowledge and Openness
to Truth

Courage and Caution

Love of Self
and Others

Dynamics of Mature Spirituality

Ignorance, Illusion, and
Closed Mind

Excessive Fear or
Lack of Caution

Narcissism,
Egoism, Hate

Dynamics of Religious Fanaticism

Healthy spirituality enlightens the mind by broadening the vision; it changes the heart for the better—to be more courageous and prudent—and transforms the will to be genuinely loving. On the other hand, unhealthy religiosity darkens the mind by narrowing the vision, hardens the heart with fear and foolhardiness, and transforms the will to be selfish and hateful in general, or at least towards people with a different belief system.

Religion is ultimately an individual matter although group influence is a strong factor. Everybody belonging to a rather fanatic group may not be quite fanatic. Similarly, everybody belonging to what may be considered a healthy denomination or branch of religion is not necessarily on the spiritually mature side. Often both dynamics can be seen in the same denomination. For example, in the Catholic church the spirit of the Vatican II Council of Bishops in the sixties (which attempted to "shake off the dust of empire" in the words of Pope John XXIII) is clearly on the healthy side of the religious spectrum. Yet there are many religious fanatics among Catholics.

In the religious life of any person, any of the three dynamic factors may be relatively stronger or weaker. Thus one spiritually mature person may be strongest in love, while another is strongest in wisdom, and a third in courage/caution. Likewise one religious fanatic may be more egoistic, another more narcissistic, and a third one more filled with fear. However, these dynamic factors interact closely, and the problems in one dynamic factor often entail some problems in the other factors as well.

Both the spiritually mature and the fanatically religious individuals can be subclassified based on their most outstanding dynamics. For example we may note hatefilled fanatics, egoistic fanatics, narcissistic fanatics, scared fanatics, and so on. I will be using the term religious fanatic, however, to mean a person who is at any of the negative extremes of religion.

Although there are many ways to view the healthy and unhealthy aspects of religion, I believe the most useful standpoint is based on the human dynamics of love, fear, and knowledge. Such a perspective will not only further our understanding of religion but also enhance our knowledge of individual and group dynamics in general.

3. MATURE SPIRITUALITY

"Out of the fulness of life shall you bring forth your religion; only then will you be blessed.' '

— Carl Jung

". . . the fruit of the spirit is love, joy, peace, patient endurance, kindness, generosity, faith, mildness, and chastity. Against such there is no law!' '

— St. Paul (Galatians 5:22-23)

The spiritually mature person shows authenticity, compassion, responsibility, discipline, self-respect, realistic sense of guilt, and cooperative/creative approaches in relationships. Spiritually mature people are not just well adjusted to their cultures; they transcend the cultural barriers. Such people show depth in their understanding, interests, relationships, and priorities in life. For the same reason, they follow the spirit rather than the letter of the laws and traditions of their religions. These ideas have found expression and support in religion, psychiatry, philosophy, and literature. We will examine some of these and the psychological dynamics underlying mature spirituality.

In general, psychiatry/psychology shuns the spiritual aspect of man. In fact, most practitioners in the field seem to either deny the spiritual or treat it with extreme caution. There have been brave souls however—James, Jung, Frankl, Menninger, and Jaspers, to name a few—who gave great importance to the spiritual aspect of our lives. On the religious side there has been—and still is—a tendency to downplay the physical and psychological aspects of human life. Here again the great spiritual leaders of East and West do emphasize holistic growth—growth of body, mind, and spirit. For even if the spiritually mature person is "not of this world," he or she is "in this world" and therefore has to meet psychological and physical needs appropriately.

It is very important to note that the fruits of the spirit listed by Saint Paul are observable human qualities. So we can judge the tree by its fruits. If the fruits had been other-worldly, such as eternal salvation, then it would have made the task of judging impossible. Furthermore, St. Paul provides another list: the fruits of the flesh, consisting of envy, hatred, idolatry, sexual immorality, selfishness, and so on. Paul's two lists provide good guidelines to judge what are the healthy and unhealthy aspects of religion. The scriptures of other religions besides Paul's reveal basically the same judgments as to the fruits of the spirit and the flesh.

The holy man of Judaism is a just man—a man of compassion, integrity, and truth. Similarly in the Indian tradition, a sage is one whose thoughts, words, and deeds are consistent with truth. According to Bahai faith, the seven qualifications of the enlightened soul are knowledge, faith, steadfastness, truthfulness, uprightness, fidelity, and humility. And the Buddha's way is to do good, avoid evil, and purify one's own heart. The five constant virtues of Confucianism are benevolence, righteousness, propriety, wisdom, and sincerity. Other religions have similar concepts.

Let me share with you one of the best responses I received when I wrote to several hundred people active in religion asking for their views of what mature spirituality is. [Explain what you would consider as healthy(mature)spirituality.] "I find this is totally tied to mature human development as a whole—if one has a good self-image, a wholesome sense of responsibility for self and life, and is integrated and self-directed, warm and open to others, then the God-relationship can be healthy. But spirituality is even more than good psychology. It is acknowledging an ultimate in life that is greater than the sum of human parts, a power of Goodness, Truth, and Beauty . . . ."

Rabindranath Tagore, an Indian poet who received the Nobel Prize for Literature in 1913, was a highly spiritual person and his poems clearly reflect it. In fact, he was called "guru dev" or divine teacher. The two poems quoted below are taken from Tagore's collection of poems entitled *Gitanjali* (meaning song offerings). W. B. Yeats commented on *Gitanjali* that nothing else had stirred his blood so much in many years. I believe these two poems express the essence of mature spirituality brilliantly and beautifully. The first poem is apparently Tagore's prayerful dream for India's freedom. However, what he wished for his country is equally applicable to every individual and every group. After you read the poem, read it again substituting 'when' instead of 'where' and substituting "let everybody awake" in place of "let my country awake" in the last line to get the full meaning of how it expresses mature spirituality.

> "Where the mind is without fear and the head is
> held high;
> Where knowledge is free;
> Where the world has not been broken up into
> fragments by narrow domestic walls;

Where words come out from the depth of truth;
Where tireless striving stretches its arms toward
perfection;
Where the clear stream of reason has not lost its
way into the dreary desert sand of dead habit;
Where the mind is led forward by thee into ever-
widening thought and action—Into that heaven of
freedom, my Father, let my country awake."[1]

and

Deliverance is not for me in renunciation. I feel the
embrace of freedom in a thousand bonds of delight.
Thou ever pourest for me the fresh draught of thy
wine of various colors and fragrance, filling this
earthen vessel to the brim.
My world will light its hundred different lamps with
thy flame and place them before the altar of thy
temple. No, I will never shut the door of my senses.
The delights of sight and hearing and touch will
bear thy delight.
*Yes, all my illusions will burn into illumination of
joy, and all my desires ripen into fruits of love.*[2]
[Italics mine]

The first poem is so self-explanatory that I wish to comment only
on the line about the world broken up by narrow domestic walls.
Walls of separation can obviously exist between individuals and
between groups of people. But less apparent walls can be present
within the individual.

The world of an individual can be broken up into fragments by
various conflicts. Narrow domestic walls remind me of the
psychological defense called compartmentalization whereby the
person keeps different aspects of life in different compartments—
instead of integrating them into a healthy whole. "Sunday
Christians" and "Friday Moslems" compartmentalize their religious
life to particular days. An American Indian told me the story of an
interesting exchange between a Christian and an American Indian.
The Christian noticed the American Indian was gathering twigs for
firewood. It was on a Sunday. The Christian asked the Indian,
"Don't you know it is Sunday?" The Indian replied, "Yes, I know. So
what?" The Christian said, "You should be praying and resting on
Sunday because it is the 'Lord's day'." To that the Indian retorted,
"For me everyday is the Lord's day."

There is a useful place for compartmentalization or division of labor in everyday life. Within certain limits it is quite healthy. However, deep down there must be integration in order for us to be spiritually mature. The spokes of the wheel, while diverging at the periphery, must meet at the center. The unnecessary walls of separation between individuals, between communities, and between nations cause immense conflicts. Besides the sufferings caused by nature's vagaries, our species creates all forms of suffering for itself.

The second poem of Tagore quoted above opposes the tendency of some religious people to negate the life here on earth. The tendency to "crucify the flesh" is not healthy. What is important is to combine our passions with good direction, as Jewish philosopher Martin Buber advocated. Buber argued that good and evil are similar in nature—not diametrically opposed as often viewed. Passion is the evil urge and pure direction is the good urge. "To unite the two urges implies: to equip the absolute potency of passion with the one direction that renders it capable of great love and of great service. Thus and not otherwise can man become whole."[3] If we kill our passions, we will be sterile in more ways than one. That is not healthy spirituality.

Kahlil Gibran expressed the importance of passion and reason beautifully:

> "Your reason and your passions are the rudder
> and the sails of your seafaring soul.
>   If either your sails or your rudder be broken, you
> can but toss and drift, or else be held at a standstill
> in mid-seas.' '[4]

The dynamic factors of mature spirituality—courage, love, and wisdom—are intimately interconnected. Courage is acting on the basis of love and wisdom, taking reasonable risks. Love is nurturing oneself and others with courage and wisdom. And wisdom is a healthy balance of reason and intuition, the kind of knowledge that comes with love and courage, and is always openminded. We will look at each factor briefly here and in greater detail in subsequent chapters.

A. Courage. All great prophets and genuine mystics were men and women of courage. They stood for the truths that motivated them. Neither pain nor suffering, not even death, dissuaded them from their path of spirituality.

Courage is not foolhardiness. Caution or prudence is the other side of the coin of courage. I will be using both words—caution and prudence—interchangeably. In psychological terms, caution or prudence is a matter of healthy anxiety. Like a healthy sense of pain, a healthy level of fear or realistic anxiety protects and motivates us.

Without courage, mature love is impossible. To love deeply, one has to take risks. And it takes courage to keep an open mind. Nietzsche had observed that the courage of one's convictions is a common error; he advocated the courage to attack one's convictions. In order to use both reason and intuition, courage is essential. That is why courage and wisdom go hand in hand.

Excessive fear is obviously absent where there is courage. The two are incompatible. People whose spirituality is mature do not show excessive fear of God, or karma. On the other hand, they show caution; they do not handle poisonous snakes, drink poison, or go on starvation diets to test their faith or prove their belief. Spiritually mature people may do such deeds as handling serpents if it is for the sake of love and if it is the only wise choice available. For example, they may handle a poisonous snake to prevent it from biting someone. Since courage is guided and controlled by love and wisdom, we can understand courage better as we move on to those other two cardinal factors of mature spirituality.

B. Love. Love is the nurturing force in sentient beings. Its potential is undoubtedly greatest in our species. Mature spirituality involves genuine love of self, of others, and of God. God is understood somewhat differently by various religions. And in the case of atheistic Buddhists, instead of love of God, there is love of bodhisatwas or those who have become enlightened. When love is sidetracked and stunted, it becomes narcissism or egoism—pride and greed respectively—in religious literature. And when love is degenerated into its opposite, it becomes hate, which is even more destructive than narcissism and egoism. Pride and greed contain hate of others in their bloated bellies.

Genuine love involves a healthy sense of loyalty to one's group or community. In spiritually mature people such loyalties do exist. However, group narcissism and group egoism are not the stuff of mature spirituality. What makes courage and love possible is true knowledge or wisdom.

C. Wisdom. Right knowledge is the first of the eight-fold paths to spiritual maturity that the Buddha taught. Right knowledge and the open-mindedness to keep that process going strong is what wisdom is about. The healthy side of all religions teaches the importance of wisdom. Authentic religions accept the importance of reason as well as of doubt. Conceptual and experimental knowledge are given their proper place. New information from various sources of knowledge is viewed with an open mind by the spiritually mature individual, whereas the religious fanatic rejects outright everything that does not fit into his/her narrow world-view.

Without courage there cannot be wisdom because wisdom involves certain risks, particularly the risks of openness and love. Buddha taught that compassion is the active part of wisdom. Where there is no love and compassion, there is no real wisdom. Various issues about courage, love, and wisdom will be discussed in detail in subsequent chapters. Here I would elaborate on the highly integrated personalities that result from these three dynamic aspects working together.

Integrated Personality. Carl Jung emphasized the importance of wholeness. "Jung understood God's call to each person as a call to the realization of his or her own wholeness...."[5] He talks about two steps in the process of integration—one is individuation and the other transcendence. These two go hand in hand. In individuation, various components of the personality are expressed and not repressed. In transcendence the opposing aspects of the personality are well synthesized or harmoniously blended. Take, for example, the sexual aspects of a personality. According to Jung, every person has a masculine and a feminine side. If a man develops the masculine aspect at the expense of the feminine aspect, he becomes a macho male. Or, if his feminine side grows at the expense of his masculine side, he becomes a wimp. Incidentally, macho and wimp are popular, not Jungian, terms. A man whose masculine and feminine aspects grow and blend together transcends both parts and becomes an integrated male in his sexual role. Erik Erikson noted how Gandhi showed this quality. (See chapter on Gandhi.)

Viktor Frankl emphasized that human beings become individualized and integrated when they are centered around the spiritual core: "... only the spiritual core warrants and constitutes oneness and wholeness in man. Wholeness in this context means the integration of somatic, psychic and spiritual aspects."[6] Similarly, Karl Menninger in his interesting book, *Whatever Became of Sin?*, states that mental health includes physical, social, cultural, and spiritual health.

From an existential point of view, integrated personalities are authentic individuals who face the existential dilemmas appropriately and relate authentically and creatively in life. (More in Chapter 5.) From a psychodynamic point of view, the integrated people use mature psychological defenses such as sublimation, altruism, anticipation, and humor. (More in Appendix.)

Let me shift gears now to religious thinkers. Paul Tillich, who defined faith in terms of one's "ultimate concern," observed, "The ultimate concern gives depth, direction, and unity to all other concerns, and with them, to the whole personality."[7] He further stated that these are the qualities of being an integrated person.

Hazrat Inayat Khan, the great Sufi mystic, commended the Hindu salutation of joining the two palms and raising them up. He explained it as meaning that we evolve by unity.[8] The meaning of "religare" (Latin for religion) is to "bind together" or "unite" and the meaning of yoga in Sanskrit is "to join" or "reunite." Being born again—a spiritual rebirth, as in the Christian sense, or enlightenment in the Buddhist sense—is also indicative of a higher integration of the person.

Thomas Merton attached much importance to integration. In *New Seeds of Contemplation*, he expresses the view that spiritual life is a balanced life involving the body with its passions, the mind with its logical thinking, and the spirit which is illuminated by God, all working together to make a complete person. In another book— *Contemplation In a World of Action*—Merton deals with the importance of "final integration" more thoroughly. The idea of spiritual rebirth, notes Merton, is not just a Christian idea, but something shared by other spiritual traditions as well.

Merton utilized many ideas of psychoanalyst Reza Arasteh in discussing the whole matter of integration. Monastic life is meant to provide the environment in which higher integration can take place. A degree of disintegration and a phase of existential moratorium (anxious search and a level of detachment from social roles) precede the process of higher integration. Merton frankly expressed his opinion that monastic life may lead to growth and integration or it may provide a safe haven of escape from the world without facing the challenges of growth. He fully agreed with Arasteh's thesis that final integration involves rising above one's culture and forming a universal identity. In fact, Merton's concluding sentence in the chapter titled "Final Integration" states: "The path to final integration for the individual, and for the community, lies, in any case, beyond the dictates and programs of any culture ('Christian culture' included)."[9]

With his concern over violence, Merton emphasized that the finally integrated person is a peacemaker. This is an extremely useful point that can often help us to distinguish between the individual who is truly spiritually mature and the pretender. A genuine peacemaker is one who is willing to understand, negotiate, and work with the opponent. He/she minimizes hate and maximizes the dynamics of love. It is abundantly clear from many of Merton's writings that his ideal of the peacemaker was Gandhi.

Other spiritual leaders accept the minimum use of violence in favor of a just cause when nonviolent alternatives fail. Such violence is not motivated by greed, pride, hate, irrational fear, ignorance, or narrowness of vision.

The work of Arasteh that fascinated Merton deserves our

attention here. Arasteh, with Persian background and a deep knowledge of Sufism (the mysticism of Islam) and of Western thought, found psychoanalytic understanding of man (and woman) incomplete. He pursued his quest, influenced by writings of Sufi mystic Rumi and of psychoanalyst, social philosopher Erich Fromm, and came up with several valuable ideas which he published in his *Final Integration in the Adult Personality.*

Arasteh points out that culture transforms the individual driven by biological drives into a person controlled or guided by cultural values. That is progress, but if the person does not move further, he/she loses the potential to become fully integrated. Culture produces its own blind spots and tends to thwart further growth of the individual self. Those who pursue growth beyond cultural adaptation go through a phase of disintegration ('fana' in Sufism), purifying the heart of its unhealthy attachments and enlightening the mind on its blind spots. Then they reach the stage of final integration with a universal identity. Certainty, search for truth, and satisfaction are characteristics of final integration. Ego, Id, and Superego merge into one at this state, producing inner joy, higher awareness, and outward creativeness. Sufis refer to this state as "Baqa." Aresteh gave the examples of Rumi and of Goethe as persons who showed final integration.

In my experience, spiritually mature individuals—the highly integrated personalities—show *simplicity, depth, discipline,* and a *healthy sense of guilt* in their lives as part of their higher integration. Their communication is direct and not manipulative. And they love simplicity but not superficiality. There is a world of difference between being simple and being a simpleton—something too many clever people fail to recognize. The spiritually mature are simple but not simpletons.

Depth in life is a hallmark of mature spirituality. Such depth is evident in the inner lives and external relationships of spiritually mature individuals. The depth of their inner lives is reflected in the depth of their interests and priorities, and their deep understanding of—as well as compassion for—others. They spend time in activities that strengthen wisdom, love, and courage/ prudence. Trivial pursuits have little place in their lives except as an occasional activity for a change or as a means to a far greater purpose. The spiritually healthy are not unduly concerned about appearances, fashions, and fads. They are also less preoccupied with the external observances of rituals than they are with the deeper meaning behind the rituals.

In their relationship to others, they show depth by cooperative and creative ways of relating. In the cooperative mode of relating, there is healthy give and take; not just trade-offs, but going the extra mile. It is opposite to the adversarial approach of getting the most for oneself. In creative relationships the individuals bring out the best in others. This is a major factor in the attraction people feel towards the spiritually mature personalities. Numerous individuals active in the field of religion have expressed to me the gratitude they feel towards a mentor (spiritual guide or guru) who helped their spiritual growth. This is not unhealthy dependence or a wishful fantasy as some therapists mistakenly interpret. The really healthy mentors do not infantilise their disciples. Creatively helping someone to grow is entirely different from using one's power to control others. However, there are false gurus as there are false prophets.

In following rules and regulations of their denomination, the spiritually mature go beyond the external structure of rules and regulations to the inner meaning of the laws. They are endowed with the spirit imbedded in Jesus' saying that the Sabbath is made for man, and not the other way around. The sufis use the analogy of a walnut for religion. The shell represents the religious laws, and the kernel is symbolic of the spiritual path. The shell has a protective function but it is the kernel that is both nurturing to us and has potential for giving life to a new plant. In fact, the shell has to break at the proper time to let the new life grow forth. Even so strict a theologian as St. Augustine said, "Love God and do what you will." Such statements are not meant to negate the place for rules and regulations but to transcend the literal meaning of the laws and pursue the deeper meaning.

Depth also involves a degree of 'tragic sense' as to the sufferings of life. But it is not a total despair or hopelessness. Along with and beyond the tragic sense, the spiritually mature find a universal meaning that makes life noble and special—sacred, to borrow the religious term.

Good humor is an aspect of depth. Sarcasm may be just sugar-coated bitterness. Wit may show intellectual sharpness. But humor indicates an overall depth of personality.

Psychological mindedness is another major feature of an individual with depth. Psychological insight is very important in spiritual growth because it helps the individual to differentiate between the truly spiritual and the neurotic aspects disguised as spiritual. Great spiritual masters of all times past showed deep psychological insight. Hazrat Inayat Khan taught that psychological understanding opens the way to mystical knowledge. And he added that psychological backwardness is a reason for the blindness of man to mystical vision.

Although Sigmund Freud was critical of religion, the psychological truths Freud discovered have helped modern men and women tremendously to pursue healthy spirituality. Famous theologian Hans Kung agrees that Freud rightly criticized the church's abuse of power, wrong forms of religion, and the traditional image of God as the vindictive or kind patriarch. While Freud ignored the positive aspects of religion, Carl Jung shed light on many of those very aspects.

Mystical vision or an integrated and transcendent world view— that is, transcending the apparent reality—is also a result of depth. According to ancient Chinese and Indian wisdom, small minds see separateness of things but great minds perceive the unity of all. Because of the depth and breadth of their vision, the spiritually mature show a compassionate rather than a hateful outlook on people with other world views. And they have a willingness to surrender to the greater mystery of the universe.

Betty, one of my patients, found that her church was not helping in her spiritual growth. The minister of this church was focusing on superficial matters such as his objection to women wearing pants and teenagers listening to rock music. He spent very little time on love, compassion, integrity, and the like. Betty expressed her disappointment to the minister: "My spirituality is in my heart, not in my pants." But the minister was too stubborn to change his ways and Betty finally joined another church that suited her spirituality.

Compassion and willingness to sacrifice are also intimately related to depth. Superficial sentimentality may express much sound and fury without doing anything significant. The case of compassion is the opposite. It shows willingness to sacrifice without much ado.

Another important aspect of mature spirituality is healthy discipline—neither rigidity nor looseness. I define discipline as *beautiful behavior*. It was Tagore, I believe, who observed that beauty lies in harmonious restrictions. That is a wonderful idea. Music, poetry, a good painting, and a handsome figure are all beautiful because of an harmonious restriction of their component parts. The great Chinese master Chuang Tzu said:

> "When I make wheels,
> If I go easy, they fall apart,
> If I am too rough, they do not fit.
> If I am neither too easy nor too violent
> They come out right. The work is what
> I want it to be."[10]

Discipline involves delaying gratification, having healthy priorities, and facing the real issues of life. It also means patience and persistence. Often discipline involves doing the more difficult task first. Mark Twain reportedly advised swallowing the bigger frog first, if one has to swallow two frogs. Disciplining our instincts, wishes, and needs form important parts of spiritual training.

Spiritual exercises such as meditation, prayer, fasting, religious rituals, and yoga help people to become better disciplined.

Will power is an integral part of discipline. But will power is not just a matter of conscious determination. We need hope, wish, and positive imagination to support and strengthen the pursuit of our goals. If we don't have much hope and a strong wish to pursue our goals, then our will power remains weak. Our imagination can help or hinder will power depending on whether it is working in favor of or against our desired goal. As Mark Twain advised, if one has to swallow a frog, one shouldn't look at it for too long. One of the ways hypnosis helps to overcome a problem is by focusing the imagination on the benefits of being free from the problem. (More on the power of imagination in the chapter on Love.)

Religious fanatics also may show strong will power but it is used in the stubborn pursuit of their narrow world-view. The will power of the spiritually mature is utilized in being creatively and authentically related in life.

Unproductive or even harmful rigidities are not part of mature spirituality. Militaristic regimentation in spiritual life is a result of excessive fear and superficiality, not a sign of growth and maturity. Without healthy flexibility, the spiritual life remains stunted like the bonsai plant.

Sexuality is one of the major areas of discipline in religions. According to the Hindu concept, the threefold object of life in this world (trivarga) consists of sexual love (kama), wealth (artha), and righteousness (dharma). *Kama* and *artha* are legitimate aspirations in themselves, but these two have to be regulated by *dharma*.

While celibacy is one approach towards mature spirituality for some individuals who can handle it properly and profitably, I believe most people are better off with an appropriate expression of sexuality. What is important, here again, is discipline; that is, harmonious restriction of behavior. Harmony of sexual behavior should exist between the sexual drive and the other aspects of the individual such as his/her conscience, commitments, obligations, and so on. Similarly, there must be harmony between individual partners and between the individual and society.

People with mature spirituality show a healthy sense of guilt. Realistic guilt is based on real wrong-doings; it leads such people to repair damage if possible, and they try very hard to prevent repetition. They also show existential guilt or guilt about wasted potential. Instead of wallowing in the misery of feeling sad, mad, and bad—as people with neurotic guilt do—the spiritually mature translate negative feelings into constructive actions. Asking forgiveness is an important step in repairing damage if our guilt is due to transgressions on somebody else. Similarly, forgiving ourselves for our misdeeds is important together with correcting our mistakes.

Spiritual growth happens in stages. It is beyond the scope of this book to enter into a discussion of the stages of faith. James W. Fowler in *Stages of Faith* notes a significant correlation between an individual's developmental stage (based on ideas of Erik Erickson, Lawrence Kohlberg, and Jean Piaget) and spiritual growth. Albert Einstein observed three stages in the development of religion itself; religion of fear, moral religion, and "cosmic religious experience." For our purpose here, I would just say that many people go through a stage of confusion, a phase of "true belief" (fanatic belief), an agnostic or skeptical period, and finally a mystical or well integrated belief system.

As human beings, even the healthy ones are likely to slip from their usual healthy ways sometimes. Healthy spirituality is an ongoing process and not a one-shot deal. The spiritually mature take special care to keep the integrated personality from regressing to immaturity or degenerating into sick personality. Emphasizing the importance of a well-integrated personality, Dr. S. Radhakrishnan observed: "Integrated lives are the saved ones."[11]

As we examine the ugly face of religion in the next chapter, the beautiful face of mature spirituality will become even clearer in sharp contrast. Furthermore, as we explore the dynamic factors of healthy spirituality more deeply in subsequent chapters—and the way those dynamics worked in the lives of Merton and Gandhi—we will have a fuller understanding of mature spirituality.

4 . RELIGIOUS FANATICISM

"In law, what plea so tainted and corrupt
But, being seasoned with a gracious voice,
Obscures the show of evil? In religion,
What damned error but some sober brow
Will bless it and approve it with a text,
Hiding the grossness with fair ornament?
There is no vice so simple but assumes
Some mark of virtue on his outward parts."

— Shakespeare
(The Merchant of Venice)

We will explore fanaticism in general, fanatical tendencies in psychiatry as an example of it outside religion, various aspects of religious fanaticism, and finally the limited benefits of unhealthy religiosity.

Fanaticism in General. The word 'fanatic', derived from 'fanaticus', in Latin, means inspired by a deity. It means marked by excessive enthusiasm, an uncritical devotion. Some people think any enthusiasm about religion—even being a regular churchgoer for example—is a sign of being fanatic. A Catholic priest friend, studying in Rome, told me an interesting story of an Italian man. Someone asked the Italian man, "What is your religion?" The Italian said, "Catholic." "What church do you go to?" the person asked. The Italian replied, "I said I am a Catholic, not a fanatic." Enthusiasm and devotion can be healthy; the problem in fanaticism is the excess of enthusiasm and the irrationality of the devotion. In the words of William James, "Spiritual excitement takes pathological forms whenever other interests are too few and the intellect too narrow."[1] James emphasized that excess leads to corruption; excess involves one-sidedness or lack of balance.

Fanaticism is certainly not confined to religion. In fact, one can be fanatical about anything in life. Several features are common to all types of fanaticism. Fanatic beliefs and behaviors are pursued with rigidity, lack of openness to other possibilities, a sense of exclusiveness and absolutism, personal pride, and antagonism or hostility towards alternate views or ways. While all fanaticisms cause rigidity and limitations, religious fanaticism does much more; it tends to destroy the very heart of religion.

Erich Fromm suggested "burning ice" as a symbolism for the fanatic—representing the inner coldness and deadness and the outer excitement. Fromm argued that fanatics choose an idol, be it God, state, or church, and submit to the idol in order to compensate for the inner deadness and depression.[2]

In his interesting and popular book *The True Believer*, Eric Hoffer explores the dynamics of fanaticism. He notes several important features—the most prominent being a passionate attachment to a cause or a group. This is a way of overcoming the sense of incompleteness and insecurity. While the fanatic sees himself/herself as a staunch supporter of a cause, in reality he/she is using the cause as a support to hang on to. Hoffer argues that the sense of security is not derived from the cause but from the passionate attachment itself. Fanatics crave the assurance that they gain by total submission to an authority figure. Hoffer observed quite accurately how a fanatic of one ideology can more easily change into a fanatic of another ideology than become a moderate. [A recent example of this phenomenon is the rightwing extremist Lyndon LaRouche who was a leftist extremist many years ago.]

French existentialist philosopher and winner of the Nobel Prize for literature, Jean Paul Sartre, showed brilliant insight into fanaticism in his *Portrait of the Antisemite*. What Sartre observed in the antisemite is basically true of all fanatics. The only difference is that while the antisemite hates Jews, another kind of fanatic has his own pet object of hate.

Antisemitism is a passionate world view. Sartre gave the example of how some men suddenly lose their sexual potency when they discover their partner is Jewish. Because of their passion, the antisemites can be dangerous and intimidating to other people. One usually associates passion with love; but antisemites hate passionately. Sartre, like Hoffer, concluded that what these people really love is the passion itself.

Antisemites play several psychological games to keep up their fanaticism. For example they block out awareness that would reveal the truth. A schoolmate of Sartre kept blaming the Jews for his failure to get a scholarship. In reality, this man had performed very poorly in the qualifying exam and was nowhere close to getting the scholarship. But in his attempt to blame the Jews, he blocked out the relevant facts.

A curious aspect of antisemites is their attraction to evil. They focus too much on evil in the name of goodness, thereby revealing their true attraction to the former. Sartre knew a Protestant with a sexual perversion who got sexually excited by his indignation at women wearing bathing suits. He spent hours by pool sides watching women in bathing suits, being infuriated by the sights and enjoying every minute of it.

Why do these people choose passion over reason? They want the illusionary certainty of their belief rather than the indefinite approximation of truth. They are "attracted by the durability of the stone" in Sartre's words. They prefer their belief over reason and research and keep a closed mind, finding strength in blind beliefs. Another game they play is a false sense of pride—a sense of permanent superiority over and a contempt for the Jews.

The antisemite is a criminal at heart with sadistic tendencies. A woman antisemite who was attracted to a Polish Jew enjoyed humiliating him by allowing him to caress her shoulders and breasts and then rejecting him. Antisemites cannot stand solitude. Forever afraid of facing themselves, these people form strong ties to groups of like-minded people. Sartre concluded that what they are afraid of is not the Jews but their own conscience, change, freedom, responsibilities, instincts, and society.

Fanatical Tendencies in Psychiatry. The intention here is not to stir controversy or to wash the dirty linen of psychiatry in public, but to offer a better understanding of fanaticism. It may sound 'crazy' or appear paradoxical that the field claiming to know the faults and failures of human nature is beset with more fanatical tendencies than any other branch of medicine. Yet it is understandable why this should be so.

By some sort of modified Murphy's Law that everything that can go wrong will go wrong, wherever there is room for fanatical tendencies there will be some degree of fanaticism. The very nature of psychiatry, where many problems and treatments cannot be measured accurately and the etiology of many illnesses cannot be demonstrated by laboratory tests as in physical illnesses, provides plenty of room for disagreements, which indeed are very frequent. One can be consoled that the state of affairs would have been much worse without the understanding that psychiatry provides its practitioner.

The various schools of approach in psychiatry have different ways of looking at the same problem. That is fair enough. Indeed those psychiatrists who can look at the problem from different angles get a better picture of the whole rather than the ones who take one point of view only, like the proverbial blind men who tried to figure out the elephant. Fanatically behavioristic practitioners, however, tend to overlook or to play down and neglect important psychodynamic, existential, or organic factors. This is true also of other schools of psychiatry. Mind you again, fanatics are often a small minority in any group.

Fanatic psychoanalytic orientation is particularly ironic because psychoanalysts are supposed to know their defenses well and deal with them appropriately. The religiosity with which they hold their belief, the extreme reverence to Freud or another "cult" leader, the elevation of their theories to a philosophy of life, and the hostility toward those who disagree with their ideas are quite similar to religious fanaticism. Such individuals can interpret a great many things in life by the libido theory or one of the other theories.

Paintings have been interpreted as the sublimation of smearing feces; organ music viewed as the sublimation of passing gas. Surgeons are supposedly in their profession because of castration anxiety (no tinge of jealousy here, of course!).Buddhist meditation was interpreted as artificial catatonia (an extremely regressed state). How enlightening! Goethe's love of nature was seen as evidence of homosexual tendencies. Cancer has been considered the phenomenon of cells committing suicide. One can imagine how a communist might take a similar approach and interpret cancer as free enterprise by a group of cells! Poetic imagination can be interesting in itself without fanaticism. For example, take the view of menstruation as the weeping of the unfulfilled uterus. Shakespeare said that poets, lovers, and lunatics are full of imagination. Take your pick (in understanding these folks).

In *Beyond Freedom and Dignity*, B. F. Skinner provides a good example of fanatical traits in behavioral psychology. For Skinner, our belief in freedom and human dignity is the big stumbling block in our way to scientific progress. He is scornful of the idea of human autonomy. Rollo May compared Skinner to Dostoevsky's Grand Inquisitor. Freedom is the enemy of both; Skinner denies the very existence of freedom while the Inquisitor admits its existence only to claim it as dangerous for the public.[3]

Actually, a healthy eclecticism in psychiatry is far more prevalent than ecumenism in religion. Ultimately, fanatical trends in psychiatry just show a human tendency arising out of the same factors that cause religious fanaticism. As psychiatry has grown older and wiser, the fanatical tendencies have become far less than before. Similarly, a professor of religion once told me that many religious denominations became less militant and exclusive with time and with better exposure to other world views. That is not always true, though. Fanatical trends in the Catholic church reached their peak in the Middle Ages after centuries of existence and exposure to other world views.

Religious Fanaticism. Wayne E. Oates, a pioneer in pastoral counseling, noted several features of unhealthy religiosity in his book *When Religion Gets Sick.* Sick religion shows a lack of self-criticism, absence of genuine humility, presence of magical thinking and self-centeredness, legalistic morality, inability to deal with ambiguities and unpredictabilities, and a tendency to throw too much responsibility on God. All these and more are involved in an unhealthy religiosity that peaks in religious fanaticism. Let us first look at fundamentalism.

Fundamentalism. The words 'fundamentalism' and 'fanaticism' are used interchangeably. That is incorrect. Strictly speaking, only Christianity has fundamentalism. Fundamentalism is a Christian movement in America which took shape in the 1910's and 20's—a movement against the influence of modernism. Some of its roots go down to millennarianism—the teachings of a New York farmer, William Miller, who predicted the second coming of Jesus in or before 1843. The basic tenets of Fundamentalism are: literal inerrancy of the Bible, deity and virgin birth of Jesus, literal resurrection and second coming of Jesus, and the belief that Jesus's death on the cross atoned for human sin. Groups who manifest rigid beliefs, dogmatism, exclusiveness, orthodoxy, and highly conservative sociopolitical stances in different religions are now referred to as fundamentalists. I will also use the word in this sense.

Given the above description, fundamentalism has most of the elements of fanaticism. It may or may not show the militancy, the active hatefulness and destructiveness we associate with fanaticism. According to George Marsden, fundamentalists are angry evangelicals. The religious fanatics are more than angry; they are hateful. Fundamentalism contains the smoldering fire which bursts into the ravaging flames of fanaticism under the influence of certain winds in its environment. The winds are usually those of change that give fundamentalists more power and prestige or cause them increased insecurity or hurt pride. The Islamic fundamentalism in Iran turned into fanaticism once the mullahs got political power. Thousands of Iranians got burned in that fire, which is still ravaging. Hurt pride and consequent revenge were obvious in the destructiveness of Sikh fundamentalists turned fanatics.

In *The Fundamentalist Phenomenon,* Ed Dobson, Ed Hindson, and Jerry Falwell give the features of extreme fundamentalism ('hyper-fundamentalism'): intolerance, absolutism, militancy, separatism, inflexibility, weak social emphasis, confrontation, and proclamation as against dialogue. Falwell and company admit that many characteristics of Fundamentalism become weaknesses when taken to the extreme. Such weaknesses include the lack of self-criticism, over-emphasis on external spirituality, resistance to change, excessive importance given to minor issues, authoritariansim and excessive dependence on leaders, too much concern over labels and associations, and exclusivism or the belief that they, alone, are saved. The description of 'hyper-fundamentalists' fits my definition of religious fanatics. Thus the difference between fundamentalism and fanaticism is a matter of degree—the latter being a more intense form of the former.

Interestingly, even Falwell et al. do not give a list of the strengths of fundamentalism. The strong points of fundamentalism are: clear and definite goals and ideals, strong identification with the group, dedication, discipline, and willingness to sacrifice for their beliefs. Fundamentalists with their rigid views, values, and ways provide a counterforce to the unhealthy extreme of valuelessness, confusion, and lack of group identification. Any of the above-mentioned strong points can become unhealthy depending on how it is used (for example, dedication to the wrong cause).

Many people are attracted to fundamentalism in various parts of the world because of their wish to preserve traditions and traditional identity. Many others are attracted by the warmth and emotional expression. For example, the Catholic Church in some Latin-American countries has started letting the congregation sing and clap during worship service, recognizing that such activities were attracting Catholics to fundamentalism. Fundamentalism has been gaining ground fast in Latin America in recent years.There are also people who join fundamentalistic groups because of socio-political and familial affiliations or because of simplistic answers or the hope of instant salvation.

Some people, especially some fundamentalist Christians, claim that they do not follow any religion; that theirs is a personal relationship with Jesus Christ. A religious fanatic I know closely says she is a "Jesus fanatic" and not a religious fanatic.

For a clear understanding of religious fanaticism, I will present various aspects of it under three headings: Fear, Love, and Knowledge. Of course these categories interact very closely, and it is difficult to compartmentalize them fully.

I. Fear   Religious fanatics may claim that they have healthy courage but in fact they do not. They are really driven by excessive fears of all sorts. Many of their behaviors are a result of such fears. They also show a curious lack of realistic fear, what we will refer to as caution or prudence. We will examine some important matters regarding fear here, and much more in the next chapter.

Fear of Freedom. Fear of freedom is a strong element in religious fanaticism. All types of rules and regulations are imposed by religious fanatics on themselves and on others, given a chance. Women and children are often the victims of rigid rules and regulations imposed by scared men. And of course, there are women who would support any stupidity on the part of men.

Rollo May hypothesized that dogmatism is an attempt to escape the anxiety resulting from the experience of freedom. The dogmatic individual behaves as though beliefs have to be crystallized before they evaporate into thin air.[4]

Authoritarianism and conformism are common ways of escaping the fear of freedom by submission to external forces. These ways result in the stunting of the person's growth, alienation from one's true self, and destructiveness toward self and others. Cult leaders often wield absolute authority over their followers. (See Chapter 14.)

While authoritarianism has diminished in modern times, conformism has vastly increased. The influence of mass media, together with many other factors, is an important cause of this phenomenon.

Fear of Uncertainty. As Sartre noted, there are people who cannot stand human limitations, among which, the uncertainties of life are facts to be reckoned with. Religious fanatics use various techniques to escape the fear of uncertainty. One of them is suppression of doubt, which will be discussed shortly under the section "Knowledge." Another is to believe in the absolute authority of the scriptures, in the literal meaning and accuracy of their every word. Episcopal theologian Urban Holmes argues that literalism is a modern heresy, perhaps the only one. Religious rituals can be another way of trying to control uncertainty.

Irrational and Excessive Ritualism. Boris Pasternak's description of Lara, the heroine in the novel *Dr. Zhivago*, illustrates the importance of rituals in religion. Pasternak says, "Lara was not religious. She did not believe in ritual. But sometimes, to be able to bear life, she needed the accompaniment of an inner music. She could not always compose such a music for herself. That music was God's word of life, and it was to weep over it that she went to church."[5] The fact that religion provided her the inner music that sustained her didn't make her religious in the conventional sense, although her experience manifested a deep spirituality.

Freud developed his understanding—and his misunderstanding—of religion to an extent from his observations of rituals in psychopathology, and extending these observations to apply to religious rituals. In fact, he viewed religion as a universal neurosis of the obsessive compulsive type, and he regarded the rituals of the obessive compulsive patient as a sort of private religion.

Obsessive compulsive neurosis is characterized by obsessional thoughts (thoughts that are unwanted by the individual but that intrude upon his or her thinking) and compulsive behavior. Rituals temporarily relieve the person's anxiety, but the ritual itself becomes a painful and disabling symptom. Handwashing is a common ritual. It is a symbolic attempt to purify oneself of one's guilt—washing away one's sin as it were. The sufferer is often unaware of the reason for the guilt. Remember the handwashing rituals of Lady Macbeth suffering from unbearable guilt. The ambitious 'iron lady' who had believed whatever done was done and you just enjoy the spoils of victory had come to realize that "what's done cannot be undone." Although she confessed that "all the perfumes of Arabia will not sweeten this little hand," her handwashing rituals continued as though subconsciously she perceived her guilt could be washed away.

Erich Fromm showed that rituals are not necessarily a sign of sickness. He observed that there are rational rituals. The basic difference between the rational and the irrational rituals lies in their function. The rational rituals express the healthy striving of individuals and groups. For example, the religious ritual of washing can be a rational ritual expressive of an inner wish for purity. Other examples of rational rituals are fasting, marriage ceremonies, practice of meditation, and so on.

Irrational religious rituals do not express healthy striving but are attempts to ward off repressed impulses. How do we distinguish the irrational rituals from the rational ones? The litmus test is to check the fear that is produced in the individual when the ritual is violated in any way. Irrational rituals produce excessive fear, but the rational rituals do not.[6]

There is also another side to fanatic ritualism—to impress others. The worse the inner emptiness, the more the pretenses to goodness by ritualism and other ways of showing off.

Fear of How They Appear. Along with many other superficialities, people with unhealthy religiosity attach more importance to appearing proper according to their beliefs. It is not that appearance has no importance. The problem is when appearance becomes more important than the reality underneath it.

One of George Bernard Shaw's characters said "He is a gentleman, look at **his** boots." Indeed, isn't it true? Especially in the age of salesmanship! Religious fanatics tend to attach extreme importance to appearing right. Keeping up impressions is much more important to them than being true to the deeper principles. Hating and trying to destroy others is fine so long as one preaches love. Telling a half truth which gives a totally false impression to the listener is not at all wrong so long as one doesn't use a swear word or one of the dirty words. Appearance of openness is more important than genuineness. Concern over petty details of a ritual or custom can lead to hatred and violence.

Keeping the behavior of others in line is an important duty for the religious fanatic. The behavior of women and children is particularly scrutinized and kept in line. The fear of equal status for women is often present in fanatics of both sexes. By keeping women and children in traditional lines, continuation of the pattern into the future is attempted. As for men, the ideas that "boys are boys" or similar notions give some loopholes for selfish behavior.

One of the big problems that many unsuspecting people face is how to differentiate the genuinely spiritual person from the fanatically religious. Appearance can be very deceptive. Religious fanatics are often wolves in sheep's clothing. Indeed their effectiveness derives partly from deceptive appearances. Jim Jones wouldn't have been successful but for the appearance of humanitarianism and genuine Christian ideals that he seemed to follow. The serpent has to appear genuinely interested in the welfare and progress of the Adams and Eves of this world to be able to sell poisonous apples. Half truth can be the most effective lie, as manipulators of public opinion know so well.

Fear of Conscience. Religious fanatics often have legalistic consciences which are rigid and harsh according to the point of the law, but provide various loopholes. Their consciences are not based on the spirit of love of self and others, and the regret over wronging others or oneself. The legalistic conscience produces neurotic guilt— excessive fear of punishment and self-hate for relatively small infringements.

Some fanatics feel guilty for even a fleeting thought or passing fantasy upon which they have no plan or intent to act. I have seen many such cases where the person has terrible self-hate (self-contempt) and fear of damnation for a passing sexual thought which any normal human being would have now and then. Some believe thinking and doing is the same when it comes to sinning. But these same people often have no prick of conscience in being hateful to people with a different belief system.

The way legalistic consciences find loopholes is interesting. There are people who practice coitus by friction of the penis between the woman's legs (without the penis touching the vagina) and feel that they are not doing anything wrong. If the man should enter the vagina in the same situation, he would feel terribly guilty. Pregnancies have happened (including virgin births) from such practices. A Catholic gynecologist who believes tubal ligation sinful may do a hysterectomy basically for the same purpose by stretching the indication for hysterectomy and feel no guilt.

An industrialist may set up a factory knowing that the potential hazard of the chemical by-products has a good chance of producing cancer and death to innocent residents of the area. He may be a religous fanatic and feel no guilt because he is not directly killing anybody. A spiritually mature individual will feel guilty under such circumstances.

A senior psychiatrist colleague expressed amazement at the number of fundamentalist Christians he has seen who commit various sins with no sense of gullt so long as they repeat their beliefs in fundamentalistic dogmas. He was surprised by their ability to compartmentalize—put their faith in one compartment and contradictory actions in another.

Spiritually healthy people are sincerely concerned about their motivation and the consequences of their actions on others and themselves. They are not primarily concerned about whether their action can be fitted in the right legalistic mold to prevent God's punishment or bad karma.

Fear of Instincts. Fear of instincts is strong among people with unhealthy religiosity. Consequently they deny, repress, suppress, or hate parts of themselves. In the words of some Christians, they try to "crucify the flesh." In trying to control the instincts, ascetical practices are followed by various people. Some fear sexuality far more than aggression. Some fear anger and repress it only to become more resentful.

Fear of Life and Fear of Death. There are many other fears that fanatics feed on. In a way, many are afraid of life because they *may* sin; and they are afraid to die because they *may have* sinned. This can lead to physical and moral hypochondria. One such patient I have been treating for a while has shown significant progress since we started dealing with these fears based on his unhealthy religiosity.

Fears lead to excessive need for control and use of force. Religious fanatics tend to project their own dynamics of fear onto others and to believe that others will behave properly only from fear.

Use of Control and Force. Fanatics believe in the use of overt and covert force. If we look at the obvious religious trouble-spots in the world, we can see that various religious groups' use of violence, militarism and religious fanaticism often go hand-in-hand and support each other. Militants give more power and glory to the fanatical side of religion, and religion gives immoral 'moral-support' to the militants to commit atrocities without feelings of guilt or shame. This is the basis for Bertrand Russell's objection to religion on moral grounds. Without religious sanctions and prompting, most of the people in these trouble spots who maim and burn and kill their brethren might have hesitated to do it.

Their belief in the use of control and force is not confined to overt mlitarism. It is very deep and very extensive: it involves every relationship. One minister recommended paddling, in sophisticated language, saying "Apply the board of education to the seat of learning." It is not an issue of spanking or not spanking a child. The problem is the ultimate belief in the power of fear and force. The same minister didn't say anything about love, understanding, care, or any of the other aspects of bringing up children. He seemed to feel that fear of God and fear of the rod would make Jack a good boy.

William James noted that a saintly temper is a moral temper and that can mean a cruel temper. He remarked that a David does not differentiate between his own enemies and God's enemies. James pointed out how Catherine of Siena stopped the fights between Christians by launching a crusade against Turks; Luther kept silent over the torture of Anabaptists, and Cromwell praised the Lord for assistance in the execution of enemies.[7] Many of the religious cults, like the Moonies and Hare Krishna movements, have remarkable control over their members. Tremendous psychological pressure is used to make members conform.

Lack of Courage. Unhealthy religiosity does not help people to be courageous like mature spirituality does. Genuine courage comes from true love and wisdom, both of which are lacking in the fanatical side of religion. It is because of the lack of courage that people crave for the illusory certainties of dogmatism and absolutism. For the same reason they show execessive dependence on authority.

Lack of Caution or Prudence. Prudence is indeed the better part of valor. Foolhardiness is not courage at all. Religious fanatics show lack of realistic fears. People who handle poisonous snakes, drink poison, beat up themselves, cut off parts of their body and the like in the name of religion are showing lack of prudence.

II. Love. Religious fanatics may preach love but often they practice hate—self-hate and/or hate of others. When they love, it is often a narcissistic or egoistic type of love of themselves and their group.

Self-Hate. Self-hate is rather common in unhealthy religiosity. Following the particular religious denomination's rituals and rules neutralizes part of the self-hate. Therefore, if these individuals fail to follow the dictates of the religious group, their self-hate intensifies. Self-hate leads to behaviors that prevent growth and promote destructiveness toward oneself and others. It may involve hatred of one's body. Self-flagellation was popular with some Christian penitents is the middle ages. Many Moslems still practice it.

Hatred of Others. Unhealthy religiosity leads people to reject everybody who is not with their particular group. This rejection has varying degrees of hostility. The worse the unhealthy religiosity is, the more intense the hatred of others. Religious fanatics would love to see everyone else either converted or destroyed. The effect of such hatred is obvious in the religious conflicts going on in various parts of the world.

Group Narcissism and Egoism. There is a strong sense of attachment or clannishness among members of any fanatic group. That applies very well to religious fanatics. It is really a process of group narcissism and group egoism. Just as a narcissistic person is proud of self and contemptuous of others, the narcissistic group is proud of itself and contemptuous of people outside its group— especially the ones whose beliefs are quite different.

Also, just as the egoist is greedy for himself/herself, the egoism of fanatical groups shows a group greed. Often with the sanctions and promptings of their religious leaders, the group can exploit others with no sense of guilt.

III. Knowlege

Rigidity and Lack of Openness. In the words of anthropologist Westen LaBarre, any kind of fundamentalism is an "intellectual lobotomy." Fanatics hold onto their views rigidly. They lack confidence in their beliefs; at the same time, they claim complete confidence. Shakespeare noted centuries ago the connection between excessive outward show and inward deficiency—the dynamics of protesting too much.

When new information becomes available, fanatics tend to reject it outright if the information doesn't fit with their rigid views. Ideas of Darwin, Freud, and others were rejected outright by religious fanatics. On the other hand, people with mature spirituality were able to process such ideas, take what parts they felt to be true, and reject only those parts that were felt not to be true after open consideration. Mature spirituality allows people to hold certain ideas in suspense, of being uncertain whether right or wrong, without feeling guilty or anxious. They accept human limitations and believe that their God is compassionate enough to accept these.

Suppression of Doubt. Fanatical thinking opposes doubts and questions about the particular belief or ideology that the person is trying to follow. Doubts and questions are seen as snares of the devil or as a sign of weakness. Suppression of doubts leads to intellectual dishonesty—living in "bad faith," being alienated from one's own intellect.

Spiritually healthy people do not nourish doubt for its own sake or become paralyzed by doubt. They use doubt to advance their search for truth and more mature life. They keep in suspense or let go of the doubts that tend to block healthy living and thinking. They do so with honesty and integrity. Such process further strengthens the individual, and it shows a basic confidence in truth and in sincere striving. Allport said that mature religious sentiment is produced in the workshop of doubt.

Legalistic Approach to Morality. In the quotation from Shakespeare at the beginning of this Chapter, I deliberately included the part on law, because it applies so very aptly to legalism in religion. Joseph Fletcher noted that there are three different approaches in making moral decisions:

1. Legalistic; that is, following the letter of the law rather than the spirit.

2. Antinomian, or a law-less approach.

3. Situational ethics which tries to follow the spirit of the law in a given situation.[8]

Religious fanatics follow the legalistic approach. In fact, they tend to reject situational ethics and condemn it as antinomianism. One can sense the fear of anarchy behind the legalistic approach. Religious fanatics will tell you of all sorts of calamity and havoc that would befall society if people did not follow the laws and regulations that they advocate.

The golden rule is a basic principle of morality in all religions. However, the fanatics of all religions tend to give it very little importance in their everyday life, especially when dealing with their opponents.

Joseph Fletcher gives interesting examples of how a legalistic approach can defeat the spirit of the law. One case happened in a court of law in England. A woman had conceived a son by artificial insemination using her husband's semen because he had a sexual dysfunction at the time. The court decided the child was born out of wedlock and so a bastard because the couple's marriage was not "consummated."

Dogmatism and Literalism. Literal interpretation sometimes comes from fear of making a mistake or fear of the wrath of a monstrous God who metes out punishment regardless of the person's motive or integrity. Another interesting feature is the way the most self-serving of the possible literal interpretations are chosen. On one occasion a Hindu friend was arguing with a Sikh friend about some of the Sikh traditions. The Hindu, who had a strong sense of humor, said that the Sikh tradition of not cutting hair or shaving is based on the misinterpretation of what Guru Nanak had advised. He claimed that Guru Nanak told the Sikhs to take good care of their children. The word *bal* in Hindi means hair, and it is also a short form of *balak* meaning boy or *balika* meaning girl. So the Hindu friend claimed that Sikhs misinterpreted the advice to "take care of children" to mean "take care of hair." The argument is fallacious as far as the Sikh tradition is concerned, but the underlying issue of distorted interpretations in religion is very true of the fanatical approach.

Another example is an experience I had with a fanatic Christian minister. We were talking about different religions. He claimed to know a good deal about them. While talking about Hinduism he said he could easily prove Lord Krishna has no divine qualities but has satanic qualities. He asked me whether Krishna isn't supposed to have a black complexion. I said not really black, but blue as the color of skies and oceans. He didn't accept that clarification, but proceeded to prove his point. Turning the pages of his Bible he pointed out to me the passage which says "God is Light." "There, you see," he said, "God is light and since Krishna is dark, he is not God. He is the opposite—the devil." But I protested that the passage in the Bible was not talking about the color of skin. However, the minister just stuck to his opinion.

Simplistic Thinking. Religious fanatics often have a simplistic outlook on complex issues. They often see everything in black-and-white terms and do not recognize grey areas. They claim to have simple solutions to even extremely complicated situations. For example, a prominent television evangelist has an easy solution to the international problems: America should build more weapons, cut off diplomatic relations with the Soviet Union, and remove the United Nations from United States soil.

Along with this comes a tendency to pick one negative aspect of some movement or ideology and just dump the whole thing as evil. Theories of evolution and the philosophy of existentialism are often dumped as evil, satanic forces, or just plain foolishness.

Reading or hearing some passing comment or superficial information about one prominent leader in a complex movement is often enough for a fanatic to jump to conclusions. For example, the name of Sartre is easily associated with existentialism. Since Sartre was a supporter of left-wing politics in France, the whole of existential thinking is considered by many as communist thinking.

Two religious fanatics from two different religions gave me the same reason for denouncing existentialism. They had not read any original writings on existential philosophy, literature, or psychology. In fact, they didn't even know about any of the writers who are considered existentialists except Sartre. At the same time, both of the fanatic gentlemen were cocksure about what they believed on the subject. When I asked them why they didn't care to learn more on the subject, they said it would only be a waste of time as they could profit more from rereading their respective holy books. They also expressed concern about the sad state of my soul which was so confused as to look into something like existentialism before deciding it is just plain trash. They pitied my naive and erroneous way of wasting time. They hinted at the source of my problem as not being in the grace of God and as bad karma respectively.

Anti-intellectualism is often admired and encouraged by religious fanatics. They enjoy making fun of the elite and glorify themselves as the down-to-earth realists with their feet on the ground and their head screwed on right. The intellectuals with their heads in the clouds are such fools in comparison. You hear of the clever little schoolboy (preferably in enemy territory) who asks the brilliant question of the silly humanist professor and exposes the folly of the elite. There are farmers, no doubt, who can take swinging digs at foolish theologians and intellectuals with clever one-liners.

Benefits of Unhealthy Religiosity. Before ending the chapter on religious fanaticism, it is important to examine the benefits of unhealthy religiosity. "The idea that something is better than nothing is applicable to religion except for fanaticism. When it comes to fanaticism, the apt saying is 'no religion is better than bad religion'," said a spiritual teacher.

Apart from the natural developmental stages of immaturity before adulthood, any adult may go through a stage of unhealthy religiosity along the fundamentalistic (or even the fanatical) lines in the process of spiritual growth. It is only a transient phase in healthy cases. Many of the spiritually mature individuals I personally know have gone through such a stage. A well-respected Methodist minister admitted how he used to be rigid, moralistic, and antagonistic about faiths other than his own early in his adult life. In his case, during seminary years, the examples and teachings of some of his professors changed his sick religiosity into healthy spirituality.

Then there are people whose intellectual and emotional capacities require rigid structure, simplistic ideas, and authoritarian leadership.

Such individuals benefit from relatively unhealthy religiosity. But even they do not need active fanaticism. I know many such individuals who have given up worse ways of living (alcoholism, philandering, etc.) and become fundamentalists of various faiths. There are many elements of healthy spirituality also in their lives.

Antisocial personalities or criminals lack a sense of guilt, prudence, and genuine love. For these individuals, the hellfire and damnation approach of fear as well as the group pride and camaraderies of fundamentalism can be very impressive. For the same people, mature spirituality may seem too vague or too good to be true. Often they can relate to the fundamentalistic side of religion more easily.

Not too long ago a Catholic priest expressed his disappointment with jail ministries (several Christian denominations that minister to prisoners) because a lot of prisoners were getting "gung ho" on Christian fundamentalism. I explained that it is not surprising at all. In fact, the prison is one of the places where fundamentalism may be useful. The Catholic priest was at first surprised by these ideas. After a few minutes of reflection, he agreed.

Another important point is that the attempts of religious fanatics to control others do not always succeed. In fact, the effort often backfires if the victims are exposed to other ways of looking at life. Let me give an example. A Sufi gentleman whom I met in a Sufi commune in North Carolina told me that his mother was an orphan who was brought up by three different Christian denominations. Each group taught her that theirs was the only right way and everybody else was going to hell. Hearing it from three different groups, she decide that the whole thing was "a bunch of bull." She became an atheist. She brought up her son an atheist, but he slowly became curious about different religions. In his search he found Sufi teachings very attractive. He and his wife find happiness and peace as Sufis. Similarly, several members of Bahai faith (which has a strong ecumenical orientation) whom I have met in Alabama grew up in fanatic Christian families affiliated with KKK (Ku Klux Klan).

It is important to mention that many members of fundamentalistic religious groups are basically good people who have big problems, or cause trouble for others, only if their faith is threatened by internal or external factors. An ideology different from theirs is usually the external triggering agent that can set them off. Significant emotional stresses can work as internal triggering agents. As an alcoholic may be fine until he/she takes a drink, many religious fundamentalists may fare relatively well until their world-view or way of life is challenged. Even when they are not causing trouble, they are missing many of the benefits of mature spirituality.

Under the influence of charismatic leaders with fanatic tendencies, the fundamentalistic followers can become fanatical quite easily. People like Ayatollah Khomeini in Iran and Jim Jones in Guyana are examples of such leadership.

Temporary regression to fanatical level is not uncommon. Sometimes people show fanatical religiosity when they are suffering emotionally or physically. In one case, the man, Mr. S., had introduced his wife to swinging (wife swapping). Mrs. S. got so involved in it, she left her husband to have even more fun. Feeling the loss and guilt, Mr. S. became fanatically religious for a few months until he found an attractive woman to "shack up with," and then he returned to his areligious life.

The characteristics of sick religiosity—which are in sharp contrast to those of healthy spirituality—are clearly manifested in religious fanaticism as we saw here. The dynamic factors underlyng the ugly side of religion will become clearer as we explore fear, egoism, narcissism, hate, and the like in the next section. And finally the examples of Elmer Gantry, Jim Jones, and others will provide a comprehensive understanding of unhealthy religiosity.

PART TWO

THE DYNAMIC FACTORS IN DEPTH

In each of the following chapters, I first discuss the psychological factors, and then relate them to religion. This approach is taken to ensure clarity of the subject discussed.

5. FEAR AND COURAGE

Behold, the fear of the Lord, that is wisdom; and to depart from evil is understanding.

Job 28:28

The great virtue in life is real courage, that knows how to face facts and live beyond them.

— D. H. Lawrence

We will examine fear and anxiety as well as courage and caution as they work in the healthy and unhealthy processes of religion.

I. Fear and Anxiety

Fear and anxiety are closely linked. Both are reactions to danger. When the danger is obvious we call it fear; when it is obscure we call it anxiety. Anxiety is caused by deep-seated fear. Both psychoanalysts and existentialists have explored the causes of anxiety in depth; the insights they developed are highly relevant to the understanding of religion. Biochemical and behavioral aspects of anxiety, while clinically important, are not relevant for our purpose here.

The idea of religion as a human invention to alleviate fear and pain is common. Bertrand Russell went further to call religion "a disease born of fear and a source of untold misery to the human race."[1] According to him, conceit and hatred along with fear are the three human impulses involved in religion. Russell further argued that religion and cruelty go together because both originate from fear. He blamed Judeo-Christian influence for the spread of intolerance in the world. Interestingly, Russell considered the superstitions of nationalism even more harmful than those of theology.

The psychophysiological changes associated with anxiety and fear prepare us for fight-or-flight responses to threats. But excessive fear and anxiety become dysfunctional. Thus, all neurosis and psychosomatic disorders are associated with excessive anxiety or with psychological defenses to reduce anxiety leading to symptoms. In personality disorders, anxiety arises from conflicts with others rather than conflicts from within one's own psyche.

Physically, pain is an important protective mechanism without which we would easily lose life and limb; fear and anxiety are similar psychologically. We hear often about excessive anxiety and fear, but rarely about the benefit of a certain normal level of both. Religion emphasizes the problem of a lack of adequate fear. Fear of God is less emphasized now than before, but it is still a major theme with religionists. Hell-fire and damnation preaching is based on the value of fear, often ignoring the damaging effect of excessive fear.

I know of a good Christian woman who has a "church phobia" caused by traumatic experiences with a hell-fire and damnation preacher. This preacher used to keep one Bible on each side of the church door and tell the people that some who crossed the doorway would be cursed by God and others would be blessed by God. While many did not take the man too seriously, this lady took it to heart and was always concerned about entering the door. Although she tried hard to be good, she—being a perfectionist of sorts—was unsure of her actions and thoughts. Her preacher had a second interesting technique to terrorize people into goodness. He declared that those who did not go up to the altar and repent of their sins would be struck dead by God. One friend of this Christian lady did not go up to the altar, and he died in an accident within a few weeks of the sermon. Since then our lady has not been able to go to church because of severe anxiety whenever she nears any church.

A. Freud's Theory of Anxiety

An understanding of anxiety along with the psychological defenses that guard against it were among Freud's most valuable contributions. Freud recognized three types of anxiety: reality anxiety, neurotic anxiety, and moral anxiety.

1. *Reality Anxiety:*

In reality anxiety, the object of fear is external, as when the individual sees another person with a weapon. In neurotic anxiety and moral anxiety, the threat is not from outside but from inside one's own psyche.

Although the phrase 'reality anxiety' seems to indicate a healthy normal reaction to external danger, that is not always the case. The cause of the anxiety is real, but the reaction to the threat may be either self-defeatingly severe or too inadequate to lead to appropriate action. If one is frozen with fear, the fight-or-flight response becomes impossible, and one is inviting more danger. Conversely, lack of appropriate fear makes the individual throw caution to the winds and take quite unnecessary risks.

2. Neurotic Anxiety:

Neurotic anxiety is caused by the fear of one's own instincts. Thus, the ego may become overwhelmed by sexual or aggressive instincts. The person experiencing neurotic anxiety is unaware of the real cause of the fear. Even when a person has the phobic type of neurotic anxiety, the phobic object or situation may not be the real cause of the fear. For example, a man with a fear of crossing long bridges was really suffering from neurotic anxiety because he was having an affair. He had to cross a long bridge to visit the woman involved. In the case of reality anxiety, we learn to cope with many dangers in everyday life by avoiding or facing them. In treating neurotic anxiety, Freud's approach was psychoanalysis to uncover hidden fears. Behavioral and hypnotic approaches have become more popular in recent times.

3. Moral Anxiety:

When the ego experiences danger from the superego or conscience, we experience moral anxiety. The superego is the internalized authority of parents or parent substitutes. What is commonly called a prick of conscience is activation of the conscience by actions or thoughts contrary to the person's value system.

Connection between religion and the above ideas.

Religion may produce too much anxiety by exaggerating potential or actual natural disasters. As someone said, preachers love pestilences as opportunities to save souls. The fear may concern another group of people, another religion, or ideology. Such fears can become intense and may lead to terribly destructive action.

Hell-fire and damnation preaching is as much about the dangers here on earth as in the hereafter. If natural disasters have become a less popular subject for such an approach, economic, social, and political disasters and threats to one's cherished ideals have become all the more popular. The fear of AIDS is currently a focus of fear. The spread of another religion or a different ideology is seen in the light of extreme calamity. For example, note the vehemence with which some Christian preachers predict doom coming from Islamic and Communist activities.

When natural disasters happen, those on the fanatic side of religion often seem to take a perverse pleasure in what they see as Divine Retribution; they have an attitude of 'I told you so' along with a sense of power. See how joyously some religious people talk about AIDS as a divine punishment to homosexuals.

Religious fanaticism may also deny appropriate fear. Fanatics may overlook realistic dangers on the basis of the power of faith, prayer, ritual, magic, and the like. There are people who refuse appropriate medical help and try faith healing instead. Taking absolutely unnecessary risk is another form of foolhardiness. The Holy Ghost people of Appalachia are a good example.

The Holy Ghost people are a Christian group that handles poisonous snakes and fire. They also drink strychnine. These practices are based on their interpretation of certain passages of the Bible (King James Version). These passages include: "And these signs shall follow them that believe;they shall take up serpents; and if they drink any deadly thing, it shall not hurt them; they shall lay hands on the sick and they shall recover." (Mark 16:17-18) These passages are taken literally — out of the general context of the Bible. The examples of Jesus' own life are forgotten in their enthusiasm for a few passages in the Bible. When Jesus worked miracles, he was moved by compassion and not by an urge to prove his power or his faith. Jesus refused the temptation of the devil to jump off the parapet of a temple, thereby rejecting unnecessary risk.

Mature spirituality helps the individual to face reality anxiety realistically without denying its threat or blowing it out of proportion. It gives the person courage to face the situation with hope and with a sense of acceptance. Faith, even fanatic faith, gives courage to act. In mature faith the courage is consistent; but in fanatic faith the courage is inconsistent because it is maintained by blocking out a great deal of awareness.

Fears of sexuality and aggression have been made severe by various religious fanatics. Victorian morality was excessively strict, unrealistic, and degrading to human dignity. Even though such extremes are out of fashion, excessive fear of sexual and aggressive instincts is often fostered by unhealthy religiosity.

One minister not long ago told his television audience how he was bothered for nearly fifty days after five minutes of casually reading something of a sexually arousing nature while waiting at a local club. Indeed, if a person had such strong reactions, he would have to be much more cautious. But of course the minister quite exaggeratedly implied that, if a man of God can be so troubled by sexual fantasy, it must necessarily trouble ordinary folks so much more.

Anger is another target for unrealistic attack by proponents of the unhealthy side of religion. This is based on a lack of understanding of human psychology. What we do with the anger can be morally right or wrong, of course. Unnecessary repression of normal sexuality and anger leads often to unhealthy inhibition and stunted growth; or the instincts may take destructive forms such as sexual perversions and suicidal or homicidal tendencies. One example is the case of Jane, who made a serious suicide attempt by deliberately wrecking her car. The car was a total wreck, but she luckily survived. In fact, she did not sustain injuries. Jane's suicide attempt was a big surprise to her family; some family members still think it was only an accident. Jane grew up believing anger was something sinful and learned to repress it. She is a caring and compassionate person, a strong individual.

Many of her relatives and friends leaned on her; and she found more meaning in life by being helpful. However, for a few years prior to the suicide attempt, one family member was making unreasonable demands on her as well as treating her unkindly. Jane tried to be nicer to this person in order to make things better, but that only made matters worse. Her repressed anger and resentment gradually grew and she pondered suicide for several months. Even in suicide she did not want to leave any sense of blame on others. Therefore, she chose to wreck her car so that her death would appear to be an accident. It took a few weeks of intensive treatment for Jane to come out of her depression, recognize her mistaken notions, and make some basic changes in her life. One of those basic changes was to learn to deal with anger in a healthy way, recognizing that it is not unchristian. Learning the difference between anger and hate (see more in Chapter 8) helped her a great deal. Mature spirituality recognizes the human drives and desires and tries to channel them in a positive direction.

The very term 'moral anxiety' indicates its connection to religion. We feel guilt and shame when we go against our value system. Every religion offers a strong value system. In reality, the religious value system is tremendously modified by other value systems that prevail in a society. A first century Christian visiting the Christian communities of today would be in for a lot of surprises about Christian values in certain communities.

On the fanatical side of religion, moral anxiety is tied up with moralism -- a legalistic kind of value system with rigid rules and some loopholes. After a religious group in Michigan disciplined a child to death, they reportedly continued to claim that it was the right thing to have done. The likes of Elmer Gantry protest too much against the very pleasures they themselves secretly enjoy. Jesus was opposed to the legalistic approach of Judaism he noticed around him, and Buddha was opposed to the Hindu moralism he had observed. However, both Christianity and Buddhism, in many instances, returned to the same kind of traditions their founders tried to reform. Professor Raja Rao, an expert on Buddhism and Hinduism, attributes the decline of Buddhism in India partly to the fact that Buddhism became too moralistic just a few centuries after Buddha's original teachings.[2]

People with mature spirituality have a consistent value system based on love, compassion, and responsibility for themselves and others, and openness to knowledge. Guilt and shame are produced by actions and intentional thoughts contrary to these values.

Religious fanatics may simply deny their guilt or shame, or project it onto the "bad guys" or the devil. A young lady (religious fanatic) who became excessively morally anxious after carrying on an affair for many months, recently quit doing it out of fear of being exposed. Then she explained the reason for her affair: "the devil made me do it." If fanatics accept the guilt and shame, they may either cleanse it with a ritual or may wallow in the misery of these negative feelings. For a person with healthy spirituality, guilt leads to regretting the wrong-doing, repairing the damage, and preventing repetition. When such a person makes use of a relgious ritual, it is done with a deeper understanding, without expecting the ritual to be a magical solution.

B. Existential Understanding of Anxiety

Professor Irvin Yalom, psychiatrist and author of *Existential Psychotherapy*, shows that we are faced with four ultimate concerns: death, freedom, isolation, and meaninglessness. Our awareness of these four existential concerns causes anxiety. Most of the ideas about existential anxiety discussed here are taken from Yalom's work. I apply these ideas to religion.

1. *Fear of Death*

St. Augustine said: "It is only in the face of death that man's self is born."

In the Hindu epic *Mahabharata* there is a beautiful scene where Dharma (which stands for duty and virtue) takes the form of a crane and tests the knowledge of Yudhisthira. One of the questions is: "What is the most wonderful of all the world's wonders?" Yudhisthira replied: "The fact that people never believe in their own death even though everyone is aware of the death of others around them." That was a wise answer.

Intellectually, we are aware of our mortality, but we prevent this knowledge from reaching deeper levels. If and when we let it reach the deeper levels, it transforms us. Leo Tolstoy illustrated this point beautifully in his short story "The Death of Ivan Ilyitch."

Ivan Ilyitch was a typical bureaucrat of his society, living only acted roles. He was admitted into a hospital with an ailment. Although he knew he was dying, he could not really grasp that fact. Of course he had learned in school, many years earlier, an example of syllogism: "Caius is a man, men are mortal, and so Caius is mortal." But he did not feel deep down that what was true for Caius was true for Ivan. He suffered terrible physical and emotional pain as he stayed in his hospital bed. He was very irritable and impatient, caring only about himself—his personality traits had become worse. His increasing misery continued day after day until just two hours before his death. Then the big change happened. "At that very moment Ivan Ilyitch had rolled into the hole, and caught sight of the light, and it was revealed to him that his life had not been what it ought to have been, but that it could be set right."[3] Then he was quiet, started listening to others, became compassionate and accepting of others and himself. This was indeed a profound spiritual growth of Ivan as he finally faced his morality. He passed away in a state of peace.

Yalom noted several healthy changes in people who have really faced the issue of death. Some of those changes are: a better order of priorities in life, an authentic sense of freedom, a better appreciation of the present moment and the elemental aspects of life, better communications with near and dear ones, and greater courage to take reasonable risks. Similar changes were noted by Raymond Moody, Jr., in his studies of people who had near-death experiences; cultivation of love and search for knowledge were the two important lessons they learned.

Several important writers such as Kierkegaard, Otto Rank, Ernest Becker, Robert Jay Lifton, Rollo May, and Paul Tillich have observed that neurotics try to defend against death anxiety by restricting or diminishing their lives. Other unhealthy results of death anxiety are: compulsive heroism, narcissism, aggression, and control. Yalom gives an example of compulsive heroism in Ernest Hemingway, who lived the life of a dare-devil, but finally committed suicide when he started losing his physical prowess.

Religion and the Awareness of Death

On the surface it would seem that the fanatical side of religion makes its members confront the issue of death and face it. There is much talk about death-related issues, certainly of life after death, the end of the world, and so on. The big question, though, is: What is the net result? Does it really produce the kind of significant personal changes that a deep realization of life's ultimate limitations produces, as we noted earlier? Religious fanatics do not show the benefits of having faced the fear of death; they do not show the loving, caring, open, peaceful, and accepting changes. On the other hand, one can notice narcissism, especially group narcissism, aggression and control, and personality constriction.

The fear of death is used by religious fanatics to force rigid conformity to group norms and to have more effective power. Militant groups are frequently an integral part of religious fanaticism. When they destroy other groups, they feel all the more powerful and glorify their patron saints or God. Their God is a paragon of nepotism in practice, although ultimately just and loving in theory. Respect for life itself and concern about environment may be absent or minimal in such people. Many religious fanatics support nuclear arms build-up *and their use beyond deterrence.*

The awareness of death and overcoming the anxiety over it by transforming one's life are basic to mature spirituality. Tagore said that death gives value to life just as the stamp on a coin gives it value. According to Thomas Merton, death brings life to its ultimate goal of perfect life.[4] Spiritually mature people show positive changes from having faced death anxiety. Living in depth and having a cosmic meaning system are the most effective ways in which they deal with death anxiety. Living in depth gives a special satisfaction in life which alleviates death anxiety. Nietzsche had observed that everything ripe is ready to die. "Ripeness is all," as the poet's wisdom declares. (Cosmic meaning systems are discussed under Religion and Meaninglessness, p. 74, below).

2. *Freedom*

For Soren Kierkegaard, man is a synthesis of freedom and necessity. And for Sartre, man is his freedom. Two basic types of human freedom were recognized by St. Augustine: Freedom Major, which is the freedom of being; and Freedom Minor, which is the freedom of doing. Freedom of doing is heavily dependent on the freedom of being, as depth psychology has consistently demonstrated. Moreover, even when external circumstances are such that the individual is deprived of the freedom of doing, the freedom of being is still present. This is illustrated beautifully by Camus in his interpretation of the Greek myth of Sisyphus, who was condemned by the gods to perpetually rolling a rock up to the top of a mountain, with it always falling back each time and Sisyphus having to go down to the bottom of the mountain and roll the stone up again.

In his attitude he did not deny or minimize his condition, nor did he use any unrealistic optimism as we are often advised to do by various sources. He acknowledged his fate heroically and with scorn. Camus concludes, "The struggle itself toward the heights is enough to fill a man's heart. One must imagine Sisyphus happy."[5]

Freedom and Responsibility

Freedom and responsibility go hand in hand. Freedom without responsibility becomes licentiousness; responsibility without freedom is impossible. Repressed instincts were the major source of psychopathology in Freud's time; in our own day a major cause of psychopathology arises from abuse of freedom and avoidance of responsibility.

People avoid responsibility in different ways: compulsiveness, displacement or denial of responsibility, and disorders of wishing and willing. Compulsive or driven behavior is often perceived by the individual as an irresistible force, as if it is something beyond the individual's responsibility; for example, compulsive sexual behavior. Displacement of responsibility is as old as Adam and Eve. Adam blamed Eve, and she blamed the serpent; only the serpent had no excuse. Denial of responsibility may take the form of pretending to be the innocent victim or the innocent victimizer.

In order to actualize ourselves, we need to be in touch with our wishes, have a perspective on priorities, and make choices and commitments regarding the wishes. Making choices and commitments seems to be increasingly difficult for people.

Not long ago I saw a successful businessman and his girl friend just a few weeks prior to the wedding they had planned. The man was panicky as the wedding date approached. He and his girlfriend had dated off and on for five years. Each time they got around to getting married, the man backed out. To force himself this time, he himself made the arrangements for the wedding. He was very sure about it for a while. But the old doubts and fears slowly cropped up and overtook his wishes to marry. His girlfriend saw the light this time and broke off with him for good. The man decided to put his energies into business and have only casual relationships.

Limits of Freedom and Responsibility

Like every good aspect of life, freedom and responsibility have their limits. For our inevitable limits, Sartre uses the term "facticity"; Ortega Y Gasset calls it "our vital design"; Rollo May and Paul Tillich use the term "destiny"; determinism is a similar concept used by many. Rollo May defined destiny as the "patterns of limits and talents that constitute the 'givens' in life."[6] He further notes that there are four different levels at which we face our destiny: cosmic level (birth and death), genetic level (gender), cultural level (value system), and circumstantial level (economic process).

When we live according to our vital design, we have the satisfaction of living authentically. Our possibilities arise from our encounters with the powers of destiny. Freedom without destiny is like a river without banks, flowing nowhere. May points out that when one refuses to accept one's destiny, one is committing hubris, the sin of pride. He is not supporting apathy, but opposing the unwillingness to accept an unalterable situation. The serenity prayer which is popular with Alcoholics Anonymous asks for the serenity to accept what cannot be changed.

Factors That Help or Hinder Freedom

Too much fear as well as lack of appropriate fear hinders freedom. A healthy awareness and concern for the consequences of one's choices and the courage to be one's genuine self enhance freedom.

Narcissism hinders the authenticity and freedom to love genuinely. Self-hate also hinders the freedom to experience, to grow and fulfill life. Genuine love of oneself and others enhances freedom by helping to transcend oneself. Knowledge and the openness to knowledge likewise improve freedom. Ignorance and illusions are among the worst enemies of freedom. Various consciousness-raising approaches help one's awareness of freedom and responsibility. Authoritarianism and dogmatism stifle freedom. Destructiveness is an abuse of freedom.

Silence and meditation play a very important role in enhancing freedom. Rollo May points out that, during the pause, we can break the chain of cause and effect and the stimulus-response cycles and provide the condition by which we experience wonder. Buddha's and Jesus' solitude and meditation of forty days were pauses during which their visions and messages were integrated.[7] The experience of numerous meditators I have interacted with, and my own experiences, have left me with no doubt about these benefits. I have also crossed upon a few people who had paid their money, bought their 'mantra', used it for a while and were disappointed that they did not get their money's worth. They had totally missed the point.

Appropriate use of freedom and responsibility leads to authenticity, compassion, forgiveness, and joy. Authenticity refers to the fact that we human beings are authors of our life, masters of our own destiny. As we experience our freedom and our limitations, the more understanding we become of the similar plights of others. Hence compassion.

Freedom without responsibility and compassion can lead to cruelty. This has been proven time and time again by politically free groups that have inhumanely exploited others economically and politically. Forgiveness, like compassion, comes naturally to the one who is genuinely free. For the authentic individual, the burden of resentment is not something to hold on to, but something to get rid of. As we leave the dead past behind and explore new frontiers and possibilities, we experience joy.

Freedom and Religion

Religious fanaticism stifles freedom and distorts responsibility; mature spirituality enhances genuine freedom and healthy responsibility. The legend of the Grand Inquisitor in Dostoevsky's *The Brothers Karamazov* illustrates this point. In the town of Seville, hundreds of heretics were burned by the order of the Church. Jesus came to Seville the day before the burning was to start. The Cardinal of the Church, the Grand Inquisitor, ordered the palace guards to put Jesus in prison. The Grand Inquisitor then visited Jesus at night and gave Jesus a long lecture on the way the Church is helping the masses by taking away their freedom.

> "We have corrected Your work and have now founded it on *miracle, mystery,* and *authority.* And men rejoice at being led like cattle again, with the terrible gift of freedom that brought them so much suffering removed from them."[8]

The Grand Inquisitor had grand plans for building a universal empire and teaching people to have their freedom by surrendering it for good to the Church authorities. The authorities would take the burden of knowledge of good and evil on themselves; all the rest of the population could just enjoy the freedom of ignorance and submission.

There are fanatical religionists who claim to be staunch supporters of political freedom, freedom of worship, freedom of private enterprise, and so on. Can we say they are opposed to freedom? Yes, deep down they, too, are highly authoritarian; their freedom has more than just a tyrannical ring to it, and they are not genuinely imbued with the spirit of freedom. They are motivated by fear, pride, and their group's narrow goals. Fanatical groups condemn those who stand for better understanding and peace with opponents.

Religious fanatics give much more importance to group activities, compared to solitude and silence. And some are opposed to meditation. Even when meditation is practiced, as in some cults that follow Eastern religions, it is often a highly structured authoritarian group activity, thereby minimizing the freedom-enhancing aspects. The individual is actively discouraged or prevented from pausing or pondering.

3. Existential Isolation

Existential isolation refers to our basic aloneness; it is a gulf between oneself and other beings and basic separation between the person and the rest of the world. It is different from social isolation (interpersonal isolation): not interacting significantly with others. Awareness of our basic aloneness can be terrifying. Fromm viewed this fear as the foremost source of anxiety. When we deal with existential isolation in the healthy way, we relate authentically to ourselves and others; we move from loneliness to solitude. Religion can help us or hinder us in this process. James Bugental gave importance to the word 'apart' in connection with our interpersonal relationships. We have to be 'a part of' and 'apart from' others.

It is curious that Yalom did not touch on the problem of alienation from one's true self. This is an important theme in existential thinking and in the writings of Fromm, Horney, and others. And it is of great significance in religion. In a way this tendency to deceive ourselves is a root cause of human evil. Martin Buber even taught that it is the particular evil that human beings introduced into the world (more in Chapter Nine). 'Living in bad faith' is one of the worst things anyone can do, according to Sartre.

Healthy Ways of Handling Existential Isolation
1. *Acceptance of Existential Isolation:*
As in the case of other unalterable aspects of life, one option is for us to recognize and accept our basic aloneness. It is quite important not to mistake existential isolation for social isolation and try to solve the problem by social activities. Meditation helps to deal with existential isolation. In a meditative state we face our aloneness in a calm, relaxed atmosphere, just as we would to desensitize any other kind of fear. As we accept and affirm our basic aloneness, we strengthen ourselves tremendously and set the stage of reaching out to others in genuinely loving relationships.

2. *Unselfish Love:*
According to Abraham Maslow, there are two types of love: one is selfish and the other unselfish. Unselfish love is non-possessive, not easily threatened; it is love for the being of the other person; it involves helping the other toward growth and self-actualization. Selfish love is the opposite. Fromm pointed out the paradox of mature love—two individuals form a unity but also keep their separateness. As Martin Buber explained, love forms a bridge between one self-being and another. Loving and affirming another being helps us to further affirm our own being and accept our aloneness.

Unhealthy Ways of Dealing with Existential Isolation: Denial and Displacement
One may deny an awareness of existential isolation by keeping busy, tiring oneself out with work and distractions, drowning one's anxieties in alcohol or drugs. The denial and displacement takes several forms:

1. *Living Through Attention From Others —*
There are people who do not face their separate existence and look for attention and affirmation from others to prove that they are alive and kicking. When somebody exists through other people's eyes, it is a burden to everyone concerned. Naturally when such a person loves, it is a selfish love. Therefore, the other person is likely to feel used and may ultimately reject the relationship.

2. *Fusion —*

One way of denying one's separate existence is through fusion with another individual or a group. Symbiotic relationships and intense groups help to submerge the individual's existential isolation. Sado-masochistic relationships are of this type. The sadist needs the masochist as much as the other way around. Fusion leaves the individual psychologically and spiritually immature. The person who is fused with somebody or something also lives with the dread of what would happen if the fusion is broken.

3. *Compulsive Sexuality —*

Authentic love and sexuality together make marital relationships beautiful. Compulsive sexuality is just the opposite; it is often used to alleviate anxiety of various origins. In compulsive sexuality one is using another—in fact, using a part of another—for one's need satisfaction. Such dehumanized sexuality, using the partner's body almost as a fetish, can happen in marriage too. In one such case, the wife pushed her husband to seek therapy because he practically raped her on several occasions when she was sleeping or when she did not want to have sex. The husband, a macho man, did not see anything wrong with what he was doing; he took it as a man's conjugal rights. He was unwilling to change and decided against therapy.

Religion and Existential Isolation

Religious fanaticism often provides groups in which the individual can fuse with others, thereby losing his or her autonomy in the supposedly holy process. Sado-masochistic relationships may be sanctified by unhealthy religiosity. Such relationships may be between husband and wife, group leader and followers, or even between the individual and God. Sometimes, religious fanatics pressure even badly battered wives to stay in the marriage. The influence of humanism has helped to reduce sado-masochistic relationships. Particularly interesting is some people's masochism towards themselves to please a God who is proclaimed as loving but deeply conceived as sadistic. For who else but a sadist would be pleased by another's masochism? Living through the eyes of others with similar beliefs occurs frequently in unhealthy religiosity. What other people think becomes more important than what one really is. There is intense anxiety about possible rejection from others of the group, especially the leaders.

Compulsive sexuality may be present in some cults like the Rajnishies, but more often compulsive tendencies manifest in following rituals and traditions. Besides all these, they miss the wonderful opportunity to move from loneliness to solitude.

Henri Nouwen in his book *Reaching Out* talks about the three movements of spiritual life, of which the first is the "movement from loneliness to solitude." Loneliness has become a common source of suffering in our time; social activities and optimistic slogans do not alleviate it. Changing from loneliness to solitude is like transforming a desert into a garden.

One doesn't have to be in some kind of desert or cave to experience and foster solitude. At the same time, some withdrawal and distancing from the distracting world around us is necessary to develop the "solitude of heart" which is an attitude, a deeper quality that is independent of physical isolation. Once this solitude is developed, with regular reinforcements, it can be maintained even in the middle of distractions.

We develop the inner sensitivity and start listening to our inner voices in our spiritual journey. Gradually we develop an inner space where we can test problems and concerns. A lonely person lacks these. In solitude the person listens to the inner self. Solitude does not lead to social withdrawal; on the contrary, it enhances one's fellowship with others.

Nouwen says, "Without the solitude of the heart, the intimacy of friendship, marriage, and community life cannot be creative. . . . without the solitude of the heart we cannot experience others as different from ourselves but only as people who can be used for the fullifillment of our own, often hidden needs."[9] Solitude increases our mutual respect and compassion. So also it increases our alertness and engagement in life. By enabling us to be in touch with our innermost being, it enhances our healing powers too.

Religion can be an alienating force or an integrating force. Gregory Baum in *Religion and Alienation* notes how young Hegel saw the Old Testament as an example of the alienating tendency of religion, and the New Testament as an integrating, unifying force dedicated to overcoming the contradictions of life through love. As Hegel saw it, the Old Testament God is a divine stranger living in His heavens ruling everything from remote control. Even when He enters the lives of people at certain moments to help them out of their predicaments, this God still remains the divine stranger. Hegel saw this as a source of alienation. Also, bad religion promotes domination, not communion and love; it creates alienation from oneself, from one's fellows, and from nature.

While the young Hegel considered religion as a source of alienation, the young Marx considered religion as a product of alienation, notes Baum. According to Marx, alienation was a result of the ills of society, mainly its unhealthy economic system. Religion also adds to further alienation. In reality, one can see that bad religion is a source as well as a product of alienation. The Bible is critical of the negative aspects of religion, such as group narcissism, hypocrisy, idolatry, legalism, and superstition. Baum points out that the critical teachings of Jesus were not used appropriately by many of his followers; instead they projected undesirable qualities onto the Pharisees and the Jews.

Mature spirituality encourages authenticity; it abhors alienation. It genuinely supports the search for Truth and is comfortable with doubts and questions. I was impressed with an introductory talk by a renowned spiritual teacher. He advised not to accept what he was going to tell us just out of respect for him. Instead he told us to listen to what he had to say, meditate on it, question it, and accept what we experienced as true—remarkably opposite to the fanatical approach of "this is the truth, either you believe and follow it, or you will go to hell."

The spiritually mature are concerned about other people's freedom also. They do not have the rationalizations of religious fanatics in dominating or exploiting other individuals, groups, or nations, in the name of God and country, race or region. In dominating and exploiting, both the victims and the victimizers are alienated from each other, and also from their own true selves. Abraham Lincoln had observed that slavery demeaned not only the slaves, but also the slave owners. Genuine prophets and mystics have been hated by fanatics because the former challenged the rationalization and hypocrisies of the latter.

4. Meaninglessness

As human beings we have a great need for meaning; a sense of meaninglessness can be devastating. The awareness of not having a concrete meaning schema leaves us to search and find our own meaning. That causes much anxiety.

Meaninglessness may lead to several problems. Among them are existential vacuum and existential neurosis. The former is characterized by feelings of boredom, lack of interest and a sense of emptiness. It may lead to existential neurosis manifesting as depression, alcoholism, delinquency, etc. Other manifestations of meaninglessness include conditions such as 'crusadism', nihilism, vegetativeness, and compulsive activity.

In crusadism an individual with a deep seated purposelessness searches out and supports all kinds of movements regardless of the aim of the movements. Nihilism involves negating the usual meanings of various aspects of life; for example, love may be seen as selfish, children may be viewed as vicious, goodness as pretense for evil. In vegetativeness the person lives an aimless life, sans meaning, interest, or enthusiasm, almost dead inside. Compulsive activity has been a recurring theme as you may have noticed. There are various causes for compulsive activity, one of which is meaninglessness.

Source of Meaning

Religon is a powerful source of meaning in life. There are also several secular sources of meaning, many of which have been influenced by religion. The important secular sources of meaning are altruism, dedication to a cause, creativity, hedonism, self-actualization, and self-transcendence.

Religion and Meaninglessness

Religion provides a cosmic or universal meaning system which often involves belief in a supreme being or creator. Belief in the soul transcending this life and in the existence of a supernatural realm is typical of religion. When religion is healthy, it provides meanings that help to integrate people, helping them to grow in courage, wisdom, and love. Altruistic, creative, self-actualizing, and self-transcending aspects of secular meaning are parts of a healthy religious meaning. The examples of spiritually mature leaders have given inspiration and meaning to the lives of millions throughout the ages.

Religious fanatics show crusadism (as in the Christian crusades of the Middle Ages), nihilism (as in the exteme life-denial of some religions), and various kinds of compulsiveness. Religious fanaticism provides a rigid, narrow, and often contradictory meaning system. Like any meaning system, it also relieves the anxiety of meaninglessness. But that benefit is gained at the expense of growth and maturity.

As the Bible teaches, it is wise to build a house on a rock, to have a strong foundation or home base. It is totally different to chain oneself to a rock. Those with mature spirituality build their home base on the bedrock of the basic principles of religion, but they leave home and explore and experience the outside world and invite others to their homes. Religious fanatics chain themselves to the rock of narrow attitudes leading to constriction and destruction.

II. Courage

The word 'courage' originated from the same root as the French word "coeur" for "heart." Courage involves firmness of heart, not the heartlessness of cruelty and destructiveness. Courage is the strength to face fear and difficulty. It has been held in high esteem by all societies. Ernest Hemingway defined it as "grace under pressure." According to Aristotle the courageous person acts for the sake of what is noble. That means courage is the affirmation of our goodness in spite of difficulties. Courage is an "affirmative answer to the shocks of existence" in the words of Kurt Goldstein. Courage always involves taking risks; where there is no risk, there is no place for courage. As the cliche puts it, "no guts, no glory." At the same time, all risktaking is not due to courage. In fact, some risktaking may be from foolhardiness. What makes the difference? That is where the factors of love and wisdom come into the picture. Risk that is motivated by love and guided by wisdom is courage. Risk taken without the guidance of wisdom and the motivation of love is either foolhardiness or bravado. Bravado involves attempts to prove one's power to oneself and others.

In other words, caution is an essential part of courage, because it protects and promotes life. In the section on love, we will see that courage is an important aspect of deep love. Ferocious actions motivated by hate may sometimes look like courage but are not really so; they are only destructiveness. Rage is not courage. The risk taken in the service of selfishness or hate is a perversion of the noble potential of courage in us.

Religion and Courage

Healthy spirituality supports courage and caution: we have already seen how it helps to face the fears arising from our existential dilemmas and from our superego and instincts. Paul Tillich, in his seminal work *The Courage To Be,* make many interesting observations about religion and courage. Although himself a theologian, Tillich had sharp psychological insight and blended his theology and psychology beautifully. He was quite aware of the way religion can create false courage which leads to neurotic limitations of self rather than self-affirmation.

Tillich says: "Pathological anxiety is the consequence of the failure of the self to take the anxiety upon itself. Pathological anxiety leads to self-affirmation on a limited, fixed, and unrealistic basis and to a compulsory defense of this basis."[10] In true courage, the self faces the anxiety and acts appropriately in spite of the anxiety. Tillich courageously observed that much courage created by religion is not true courage; it leads only to diminished being. The religious mystic, however, shows a tremendous degree of true courage in his/her self-affirmation, transcendence of the self, and identification with the ground of being. (More about the mystic's identity in Chapter 15.)

Courage helps the spiritually mature person to overcome the fears of dependence/independence, authenticity, commitment and depth. We have already dealt with most of these issues, except the fear of depth which leads to superficiality. *Religion itself may be used by many individuals as a defense against spiritual growth.* Such people often do not want to face the difficulties and stresses that accompany living in depth. Of course they also miss the benefits. In fact the great opportunity of our being human is the capacity for living in depth.

The courageous lives of prophets, religious founders, and religious reformers are among the most glorious highlights of human history. It has been said that the blood of martyrs has nursed religious movements. The reason is the courage generated in followers by the martyr's example.

An incident in the life of Martin Luther King, Jr. illustrates how religion provides courage. One night in January, 1956, in the midst of the black boycott of Montgomery city bus lines, King was afraid of threats to his life. He felt weak and had second thoughts about his fight for civil rights. He could not sleep. King prayed hard and his prayer was answered. He felt reassured of Jesus' support and went ahead with a civil rights movement that changed the history of racial relationships.

Mahabharata teaches that it is courageous to forgive. Spiritually mature people show the courage to forgive others and themselves. Individuals and groups who forgive and reconcile move on to harmony and progress.

The importance of courage is beautifully illustrated in Hindu mythology. Lord Shiva who does the cosmic dance is represented with four hands. With his upper right hand he holds a drum which is a symbol of creation. And with his lower right hand he makes a gesture (*abhaya mudra*) representing the removal of fear. Courage and creativeness go hand in hand.

The connection between creativeness and courage has been recognized for a long time. Balzac, a great writer himself, was one of those who emphasized this connection. Rollo May did the same. As we read in the chapter on Mature Spirituality, creativeness is an important accompaniment of higher integration.

Healthy integration of mature spirituality involves tremendous courage to deal with various sources of anxiety, as we noted from Freudian and existential viewpoints. Courage helps us to be in touch with our true being and to become authentic individuals. It also enables us to overcome the tendency towards selfishness, making us genuinely loving. And it facilitates our search for truth with an open mind, making us wise. Nietzsche's statement that error is cowardice is profoundly insightful. Healthy spirituality works against this error, as our examples of Gandhi and Merton in Part III will show. In the next chapter we will explore egoism and narcissism, two forms of selfishness where courage fails and fear wins.

6. NARCISSISM AND EGOISM

"If I am not for myself, who will be? And if I am only for myself, what am I?"'

— Rabbi Hillel

"The wrong asceticism torments the self; the right kind kills selfness.''

— C. S. Lewis.

The words narcissism and egoism are often used interchangeably. That is incorrect. Although both have several common characteristics, such as immaturity and self-centeredness, there are some important differences also. Erich Fromm made a point that, whereas the narcissist has a distorted view of his/her importance, the egoist may have a realistic picture in that regard. The basic problem of the egoist is greed, wanting too much for oneself.[1] Narcissism and egoism in psychology are the sins of pride and greed in religion.

Our selfishness can take the form of egoism or narcissism. We need food, shelter, a degree of control over our environment, and the like for our survival (survival of our 'phenomenal ego' to use Huxley's term—see more in Chapter 10). Taking these needs to an extreme is egoism. All sentient beings tend to enjoy pleasure and avoid pain. One can be greedy about pleasure (hedonistic) also. Apart from surviving, we also need self-respect; and taking this need to an extreme is narcissism. Self-respect is so important to us that we human beings even tend to destroy ourselves when we lose self-respect.

In my professional and personal experience as well as in reading history, I notice many more problems arising from egoism than from narcissism (egotism). In psychiatry there is a large body of literature on narcissism but hardly anything on egoism. I suspect that one of the reasons may be that the Judeo-Christian background of the authors makes them more sensitive to the problems of pride than to those of greed perhaps because the Judeo-Christian tradition emphasizes pride as the root of all evils. Possibly psychiatrists with a Buddhist background will correct the imbalance in the future.

Liberation Theology is a recent systematic Christian movement that deals with issues of greed, power, and social responsibility. One hopes it will stimulate studies on egoism.

Being admired is of utmost importance to the narcissist. For the egoist what is most important is to have more possessions, money, power, wealth, etc. If these two sick personalities have to choose between gaining name and gaining money, the narcissist would easily choose name and the egoist would, with equal ease, choose money. Similarly between power and glory, the egoist would choose the former and the narcissist would choose the latter. But then we have to recognize how power and glory overshadow. For there is power in glory and glory in power.

Egoism

Webster's Dictionary defines egoism as "excessive concern for oneself usually without exaggerated feelings of self-importance." As an example of egoism let me give the case of a physician I treated many years ago in another part of the world and about whom I knew from several sources. We will call him Dr. Grady. Dr. Grady used to speak nicely and very personably to his patients and anybody who would give him business. However, he kept his employees on their toes by his unreasonable demands. Even with his colleagues in his group he used to behave as if he had two personalities—sweet when he wanted to get something out of them and sour otherwise. In fact, he was called "sweet and sour pig," by some. He was so controlling and selfish that his colleagues had to leave him. Even when he had a huge practice he would use expressions such as "we are already starving" whenever he heard about any other physician joining the hospital staff.

He had no scruples except for being legally safe. His charts were the most legally safe charts. His authoritarianism and penetrating look made nurses and other hospital employes follow his wishes out of fear. He had no hesitation in 'stealing' patients from other physicians.

The dynamics of fear were very strong in him. When he was under a significant amount of stress from conflicts with family and colleagues, he became tense and uptight. He was also suspicious and vigilant about what others were doing. His insecurity was affecting his functioning. So he sought my help, mostly to learn relaxation techniques.

Even more interesting was the way he used to control his patients by fear. He would tell reluctant or ambivalent patients: "You are not going to make it." "This is going to kill you." "You will be in terrible shape." He was fond of putting patients in the hospital and keeping them there for a long time. To patients who did not want to go in the hospital, he would say with a stern face and piercing stare: "You should be in the hospital." He would not discuss with them alternatives, pro's and con's, etc. He got his way with most people by his scare tactics.

He did not care much about love; he wanted and demanded respect and obedience from his wife and children. Even though he was making three times the money an average physician makes, he did not support his children's higher education. He and his wife had a rather sado-masochistic relationship; he frequently threatened to divorce her. In fact, I was told he kept divorce paper in his car all the time.

Dr. Grady's problem was greed but not pride. He did not glorify himself or devalue others as a narcissist would do. He did not look down on his colleagues so much as he just wanted everything for himself, being terrified of sharing. Incidentally Dr. Grady was not interested in working on his greed; so the therapy only helped him through the crisis. He always claimed to be a good Christian. His egoism was not caused by his religion but his religion, instead of challenging the egoism, supported it. For him, any business practices that will not lead to one's incarceration were acceptable and highly desirable for a christian. He interpreted his worldly success (largely attributable to his greed) as a sign of God's blessing.

Religion and Egoism

Healthy spirituality is opposed to egoism. By promoting genuine love and compassion, the healthy process of religion prevents egoism or helps to eliminate egoism where it is present. Unhealthy religiosity on the other hand tends to promote individual, or more commonly, group egoism. There have been plenty of instances where religious leaders supported, even instigated, their followers to take over properties belonging to other religious groups. For example a Mormon Church leader Sampson Avard sanctioned his followers to rob and plunder the Gentiles and build up the kingdom of God. Colonialism, exploitation of lower class by upper class, and exploitation of lower castes by higher castes have been sanctioned, even sanctified, by religious fanatics.

One of the most interesting phenomena is the way unhealthy religiosity tends to transform egoism into narcissism. I have seen many individuals who became less greedy after joining fundamentalistic religious groups only to become more proud and arrogant on the basis of their newfound glorified image. This is like falling from the frying pan into the fire.

Narcissism
    The word 'narcissism' is derived from the Greek myth of Narcissus, a handsome young Thespian. His mother was a river nymph, and the prophet Tiresias had predicted to her that Narcissus would live to a ripe old age if he did not know himself. Echo, a beautiful mountain nymph, fell head over heels in love with Narcissus and followed him around. Narcissus rejected her and Echo, heartbroken by the rejection, pined away. Out of revenge she called upon the gods to punish Narcissus also by disappointed love. Then one day he saw his own reflection in the limpid waters of a fountain; he fell in love with his reflection and lay gazing enraptured at his image. He died of languor and turned into narcissus—a flower that grows at the edge of streams. Inability to love others was the tragic flaw in his character.
    Let me give a clinical example of narcissism. Jack, a young engineer in his mid-thirties with a narcissistic personality, came for treatment for depression. He had cut his wrist superficially as a suicide gesture. He was upset and very angry with his wife after discovering that she had gone off with another man on the weekend that Jack was away on a business trip. His wife had come with him for the appointment; she was remorseful, yet angry with Jack for his repeated belittling remarks about her.
    Jack and Jackie had been married for over ten years. He was successful in his work and prided himself over it. All through his adult life, Jack had had liaisons with several different women; many of his business trips included such escapades. His wife knew about some of these and had confronted him a few times, but he had denied the charge or brushed it aside. So their relationship had grown increasingly cold over the years. Jackie was doing well in her job as a secretary. Whenever she got a promotion or recogntion from her employer, Jack was jealous. In fact, Jack had wanted her to be just a housewife. Jackie had always been a faithful wife until the above incident happened. She had known the other man through her work and he was a lot of what Jack was not—caring, warm, appreciative of others, and not haughty. Jackie not only had a good deal of respect for him; but also she was taking revenge on Jack when she went off with this other man.
    Jack's depression improved with medication and psychotherapy. After he made Jackie feel guilty and miserable for a while, they started back into an unhappy but less turbulent relationship. Jackie was not assertive about making healthy changes in their marriage, a fact Jack found very convenient. When I suggested that Jack continue in therapy to make further changes, he declined. In fact, once the symptoms of depression were better and he felt his old control over himself and his wife, his interest in treatment melted away. Whenever we had couple's sessions, Jack was intent on putting

down his wife at every opportunity. She protested a bit but acted as a martyr at other times and finally promised him never to repeat her wrongdoing.

Jack gave an interesting picture of the kind of wife he wanted to have. He asked me to imagine a female robot with beautiful feminine physical attributes, who could be programmed to do a number of things. She would be always cheerful and enthusiastic about everything Jack did, a perpetual cheerleader, always obedient and totally pleased with him no matter what he did. Jack knew for sure that such a product, if and when Sears and K-Mart started selling it, would be the hottest selling item in the whole world. He was so self-righteous and grandiose about his wishes and ideas that he had no shade of shame in depicting such a dehumanized picture of a wife.

Narcissism involves an exaggerated sense of self-importance and a need for confirmation of that image. In the myth of Narcissus, he fell in love with his *image*. The image is very important to the narcissist even as he disregards his true self. Narcissists have an air of success and confidence. Depending on what would be impressive to the people around them, they may show a self-assured equanimity or a haughty and snobbish attitude. They can change their style like some animals change color to suit the environment. Narcissists exaggerate their talents and achievements.

Narcissist's fantasies are filled with their self-concept of beauty, brilliance, and power. Power is very important for them because deep down they feel powerless, impotent, empty. As part of their craving for 'power', they pretend to be invulnerable. This is done, as Alexander Lowen showed, by denial of feelings, particularly feelings of tenderness, sadness, and fear. Denial of feelings is a way of defending against possibility of hurt.[2] In my experience, denial of feelings has another important though unfortunate function. That is the perpetuation of hoarding, exploiting greediness without guilt or shame.

Gordon Liddy described in his book *Will* how he overcame feelings so that he could kill efficiently and without any emotion or thought. He did it by working for a neighbor who was raising chickens for the market. Liddy practiced killing the chickens more and more efficiently and finally was satisfied that he could kill "like a machine." Feelings of tenderness, compassion, or empathy make one want to give to others, to share with others.

Narcissists may show pseudosublimation. Pseudosublimation is, as the word suggests, a phony sublimation which is in reality a kind of exhibitionism. While the sexual exhibitionist flashes his penis and gains satisfaction from the shocked reaction of the victims, the charity exhibitionist flashes his wealth and gains satisfaction (and possibly more business) from showing off his wealth. After all, everything that glitters is not gold. Genuine charity begins at home, is consistent, and is not a manipulative technique; it is a result of compassion. A businessman who exploits workers and customers and then turns around and gives big sums to church or charity is an exhibitionist or is trying to relieve guilt.

Interpersonal relationships of narcissists are shallow. They are need-satisfying relationships, not genuine ones. For Jack in the case described earlier, the women he went to bed with were just female machines he manipulated masterfully, if and when he needed them. This reminds me of an unforgettable remark made by a Pediatrics Resident who was rotating through psychiatry. Talking about his interest in children outside of the hospital setting, he told me that he didn't want to have his own child; that would be too burdensome. But then there are several times a week or month when he would like to have a child for a couple of hours to play with. In fact, he told me he would like to *rent a child* at such times. I want to clarify that this young physician had no sexual perversion; it was not from any wish for sexual exploitation, but it was from the wish to prevent deeper caring and commitment that he only wanted a superficial and convenient relationship.

Overidealization and devaluation of others is another interesting feature of the narcissist. Those who serve to bolster the power and glory of the narcissist are idealized and envied. Even those people may be devalued out of envy whenever they threaten the narcissist's own sense of importance. Others in general are looked down on; this devaluation helps the narcissist to feel superior. Narcissists may go into a state of splendid isolation when other approaches fail.

Narcissist's love is turned inwards. This is unproductive love. Healthy self-affirmation does not turn inwards but extends outwards to others. And thereby nature increases possibilities for newer, better, and more entities. All this is prevented by the self-absorption of the narcissist. Moreover, as the Greek myth implied and as we see around us, it leads to destruction of oneself and others.

Narcissists are very sensitive to criticism; and they hate rejection. They react very strongly and negatively to both. When I think of the old saying "Hell hath no fury like a woman scorned," I believe it refers to a narcissistic woman. Narcissists try to destroy those who may be a threat to their narcissistic glory. For that matter, the narcissistic individual is often preoccupied with his or her closest competitor and with ways to win in the competition.

Narcissists's ideals are all "sound and fury signifying nothing." They have an apparent zeal in following whatever ideals a given society at a given time makes its standard, be it high church or low church, be it economic production or marketing, be it old fashioned chivalry or newly acclaimed chicanery. But they have no genuine commitments except to their own vanity. For them, the world is a grand stage and they take on whatever role brings acclaim. Their consciences are therefore easily corruptible.

Narcissists are filled with fears on a deeper level. They are afraid of intimacy, commitment, death, true knowledge, failure, helplessness, love, illness, impotence, insanity; in short, they are afraid of being really human.

As mentioned earlier, a feeling of personal inviolability is a strong defense against the fear of death. Thomas Merton noted that people sometimes destroy weaker individuals to prove their own power to survive. In massacres throughout history, women, children, and the elderly have been victimized by those who seek revenge and the resulting sense of strength. The vicarious thrill of watching various forms of violence on screen has become so much a part of narcissistic culture that it is considered a highly civilized activity. Many a primitive tribesman would be shocked indeed by the popularity of such entertainment. Dr. Jane Christian, Professor of Anthropology at the University of Alabama in Birmingham, confirmed this from her experience with tribesmen.

Among the worst fears of a narcissist is the fear of exposure, the fear of facing his/her true self. Therefore, in trying to keep the mask, he or she keeps on doing more and more evil. Just as the Pharaoh's heart hardened with more and more acts of evil, the narcissist gets increasingly entangled in the mesh of his own false pride and irrational fear.

Group Narcissism

The regressive quality of group dynamics has been noted by numerous writers throughout history. "The masses are asses," a common-sense notion, is based on true experiences. Nietzsche said madness is the exception in individuals but the rule in groups. The crowd that wanted to crucify Jesus and free Barabbas and the concerned citizens who decided that Socrates was too much a threat to their posterity and insisted on his death by drinking poison, are good examples.

Freud noted that emotionality, irrationality, suggestibility, thirst for illusion, and the charisma and prestige of the group leader are important factors in group psychology. He elaborated on two aspects of group dynamics; namely, identification and hypnotic effect. Freud argued that man is more a horde animal, "an individual creature in a horde led by a chief" than a herd animal, as Trotter had pronounced. The group members make the group leader their ego-ideal and identify themselves with the leader. This also leads to brotherly feelings toward others in the group. As an example, Freud pointed out how Christians love Christ as their ideal and feel a common identity with other Christians.[3] Again, just as individual narcissism is sick, so also is group narcissism. While the scope and damage caused by individual narcissism are limited, those caused by group narcissism are much more extensive. Evil individuals with personal narcissism would have been laughed out of court or put in prisons but for the group narcissism they were allowed to play with.

Scott Peck in his book on human evil, *People of the Lie,* pointed out that specialization of groups leads to fragmentation of conscience and avoidance of responsibility. Another important factor is infantilization of the followers by their dependence on the leader. Group pride, *esprit de corps,* is used as a cohesive force that binds the group. The other side of that coin is devaluation or contempt for others, especially others who are a threat to the group's existence or to its glory. Peck gives an interesting analysis of the My Lai massacre during the Vietnam War as an example of group evil. Many American soldiers were involved in killing a group of innocent villagers. But none of them took responsibility for the action.

By applying our knowledge of existential psychology, we can understand some other important aspects of group narcissism. Group process gives individuals a way of escaping existential conflicts rather than facing them and growing up as authentic individuals. By submerging themselves in group narcissism, individuals can deny freedom and responsibility; they need not agonize over choices or feel guilty about bad consequences from wrong choices. Fear of death is easily submerged in the busy activities of the group. Problems of existential isolation find pseudosolution in the fusion of the group. The search for meaning in life is cut short by the mass person because the group provides all the necessary meanings. And besides, the narcissistic group convinces its members that any other meaning given by any other source is of no value; it is all plain stupid.

Another function of group narcissism is providing artificial support for the sagging self-esteem of certain individuals. Poor members of a supposedly great class, community, or race may thus be much more intense in their group narcissism than other members who have good self-esteem on their own rights. Similarly, one can notice more prejudice and bigotry by unsuccessful members of different groups. They are catching on to whatever straws they can to prevent sinking lower into poor self-esteem. If only they had the insight, they could find healthy ways of improving self-esteem.

Narcissism, Egoism, and Religion

The sin of pride is considered by Western religions to be the basis for all evil. The pride of the angels led to their downfall and transformation into devils. Then Adam and Eve sinned because of their prideful rebellion in their vain attempt to become God. All religions teach the virtue of humility and oppose the vices of pride and greed. The term pride is used by many to denote healthy self-esteem also; therefore, let me clarify that, when I use the word pride, I mean the sin of pride and not healthy self-respect. In order to teach people humility, religions emphasize the insignificance of man compared to the greatness of God. Religious founders showed examples of humility to their followers; in spite of their superior wisdom and other qualities, they lived humble lives. Religious books give plenty of examples of how God rewards the humble and punishes the proud. Erich Fromm and Karl Menninger noted that the goal of all the great religions is to overcome one's narcissism. So far so good. However, how far have religions helped to achieve that goal? Or, in fact, have they made the problems of narcissism even worse and more vicious?

Fanatics do emphasize the sin of pride tremendously. They do glorify God immensely. In fact, they may take the idea of humility to such an extreme that it becomes humiliation. Some of them talk about humans being worms and worse; they gloat over the utter evil of human nature; they claim all honor and glory and dignity is God's and none of it whatsoever is man's. Every wrongdoing and every fleeting thought may be roundly condemned. Thus the individual is divested of his or her self-respect and thrown on the ash heaps of human helplessness, and given a sense of worthlessness. And then the broken and humiliated person is shown the way to glory, to the ultimate victory through the approaches that the particular religious group teaches. So the invitation to follow the group becomes all the more intense and irresistible. It is like starving somebody and then pointing the way to get to a feast.

The result of such manipulations is far from satisfactory, and some people remain in the state of humiliation or remain prone to going into the state of humiliation easily. Others develop a new narcissism in which belonging to the particular religious sect becomes the source of tremendous pride. Narcissism that is molded and sanctified by religion is far worse than the usual kind because it negates the shame and guilt the individual may otherwise feel. Hence the viciousness of religious fanatics.

Erich Fromm cited the Roman Catholic Church as an example of narcissism and its opposite forces working within the same group.

On the side of humility are the beliefs in the universality (or catholicity) of the Church, the supremacy of God, and the brotherhood of man. On the side of narcissism, Fromm cited such concepts as the Catholic church as the sole source of salvation and the Pope as the vicar of Christ on earth. In the fifteenth and sixteenth centuries, Christianity had many great humanists (I would say men of spiritual maturity) such as Nicholas of Cusa, Erasmus, and Thomas More, who stood for human dignity, brotherhood, and religious tolerance. On the other side of the spectrum, many in the officialdoms of churches led or supported religious persecutions.[4]

Self-humiliation based on sick religiosity can be one of the major factors for chronic depression in some individuals. The most chronically and severely depressed patient I have ever treated had told me a thousand times "I am no good." Her anguished cry of being no good is based on the idea popularized in certain Christian circles that if you are really good, God will bless you with material success in this world as well as with all the blessings in the other world. She had not been successful, so she felt condemned.

All the therapeutic approaches I had used and, as I understand, numerous other therapists had used, had only minimal effect. As I was racking my brain and asking some friends for any suggestions, one day I noticed she was reading the book *Compassion* by Mathew Fox. It was a big relief for me. Since then I have encouraged her to read similar books and progress along spiritual lines. Although she still has problems, her self-depreciation is less and her depression is improved. A young campus minister who worked with her for a while had introduced her to the spiritually healthy side of Christianity and that paved the way for change.

I have also observed rich and successful people whose pride and arrogance is really "out of this world" because they take their success as proof of their special connection with the Almighty.

Group narcissism of national and racial types has found favor with religious fanatics. In fact, if we look at the areas of religious conflicts all over the world, we can see it is the unhealthy religiosity that sanctifies the group narcissism and group egoism behind the conflicts. Mature spirituality, on the other hand, tries to bring understanding to relieve the suffering and improve the lot of the afflicted. While fanatic Protestants and the IRA fight viciously in Northern Ireland, genuinely spiritual Christians have been trying for peace.

Healthy spirituality helps to improve people's self-esteem and, at the same time, to prevent it from becoming narcissistic. All religious founders helped the weak, innocent, and downtrodden to gain a sense of self-respect. Acceptance by those great men meant much to their followers, many of whom were outcasts of society. Jesus raised the self-esteem of the sick and the sinners, and He confronted the narcissism of the Pharisees and the egoism of people who used religion for monetary gain.

The one occasion where Jesus used some degree of force without violence was with the people who were buying and selling in the temple. It was as though He knew that they would respond only if they knew that He meant business. Egoism or economic vested interest may be one cause for heavy resistance to change. When a woman wanted to anoint his feet, Jesus allowed her to do so over the objections of some of his followers. It was Jesus' way of accepting and affirming the poor woman; it was not for his self-glorification.

Gandhi lived a simple life to identify with ordinary Indians. That helped the Indians to identify with Gandhi and gain a self-esteem which they had lost long ago, along with their traditional trades and relative prosperity. Prophet Mohammed helped the weak, the wretched, and the women of his time to gain self-respect and respect from others. The inspirations of Buddha, Confucius, Lao Tse, Moses, and other great personalities of religion have been the backbone of the self-esteem of millions of people. Yet distorted versions of the teachings of these same great individuals have broken the back of the self-esteem of millions of others who felt even more worthless, hopeless, and condemned.

A leader of an Eastern Orthodox Church said a few years ago that it is too petty a God who cannot let human beings have a sense of dignity. That is an interesting point. The God of the religious fanatic doing everything just for His own glory and filled with wrath for any little infringement is a narcissistic God. It is the elaborate projection of the narcissist's own psyche. Buddha taught people to save themselves, and Jesus told the healed that their faith healed them. Why should we think that God cannot give the devil his due, whatever tiny due it may be?

Mature spirituality rises above individual and group narcissism. That is a major reason why narcissistic groups try to destroy mature spirituality. Mystics and prophets were victims of narcissistic political and social groups throughout the ages.

On the other hand, political and religious narcissism can go hand-in-hand, as the Catholic Church demonstrated for centuries as the religion of the Papal States. In our times we see how the fanatical side of religion supports national pride and greed. Many Christian Fundamentalists consider America as God's Country. Many of them claimed that God did not want the U. S. to give the control of the Panama Canal to Panama. Similarly, Islamic Fundamentalism in Iran and Jewish Fundamentalism in Israel foster national pride and greed.

In 1965 Pope Paul told the United Nations Assembly how

important humility was. He said, "No matter how justified it may appear, pride provokes tension and struggles for prestige, domination, colonialism, and egoism. In a word, *pride shatters brotherhood.*" How beautifully put and deeply true!

Healthy religion promotes compassion and altruism. It inculcates the sacrifice of selfish interests and discourages both individual and communal greed. Numerous charitable activities are pursued by varied religious groups. Even fanatical groups exhibit some of these positive qualities within the scope of their membership.

Let me close this chapter with some extremely relevant statements by Reinhold Niebuhr:

"Collective pride is . . . man's last and, in some respects, most pathetic effort, to deny the determinate and contingent character of his existence; the very essence of human sin is in it. This form of human sin is also most fruitful of human guilt, that is, of objective, social and historical evil."[6]

"Prophetic religion had its very inception in a conflict with national self-deification. Beginning with Amos, all the great Hebrew prophets challenged the simple identification between God and the nation in its exclusive relation to God . . ."[7]

The tendency to protect one's self and self-esteem need not go to extremes and result in egoism or narcissism. Instead it can be balanced and result in healthy love, and religion can play a pivotal role in promoting it as we will see in the next chapter.

7. LOVE

"Love is a Way to truth, to Knowledge, to Action."

— Rauf Mazari

"Love alone is capable of uniting living beings in such a way as to complete and fulfill them, for it alone takes them and joins them by what is deepest in themselves." [1]

— Teilhard de Chardin

Gordon Allport frankly admitted that religion is superior to psychotherapy in meeting the affiliative needs of human beings. Surprisingly, not much is written about love in the whole field of mental health compared to the voluminous writings on sex. My psychiatric dictionary says that love is pleasure, explaining this idea further with no reference to affection, tenderness, concern, commitment and the like! However, there are some good writings on love in psychiatry. Love almost defies definition. Two definitions that I like are as follows:

> "Love is the active concern for the life and the growth of that which we love." [2] — Erich Fromm

> "The will to extend one's self for the purpose of nurturing one's own or another's spiritual growth." [3] — Scott Peck

These definitions are still not the whole truth. So, let us break the complex experience into component aspects in order to understand it better. Since love is the word used to denote everything from a generally caring attitude toward others to the most intimate love relationships, we will look at the experience under two headings:

(1) Love in general—the basic elements of all kinds of love including love of one's enemies.

(2) Deep love. These two are not watertight compartments, but a continuum.

I. Love in General

According to Erich Fromm, the basic elements of love are care, responsibility, respect, and knowledge. For the purpose of our discussion, we cover these elements in a modified sequence — knowledge, care, respect, and responsibility.

A. Knowledge

Some Hindu sages say that perfect love is perfect knowledge. It is our greater capacity to know ourselves and others that is behind the human capacity to love intensely. The phrase "carnal knowledge" indicates, in its own crude way, the relationship between love and knowledge. The Hebrew word "jadoah" means knowledge and also sexual intercourse. Love is indeed penetrating knowledge.

Knowledge, like love, begins with ourselves and extends toward others. And it forms a circle as we accept other people's love. Realistic and deep knowledge involves knowledge of one another's strength and weakness. Jesus pointed out the problem of biased perception, the folly of looking for the mote in another's eye while overlooking the beam in one's own eye. In the passionate outlook of rosy romantic experience, the tendency is to see only the strength and to see it magnified. And then, as the reality of the negative aspects hits the romantic lover in the face, either the honeymoon ends or a more stable relationship begins.

Compassion arises from the understanding of our weaknesses, vulnerabilities, and limitations. We ourselves learn to experience our weakness with a loving rather than a hating attitude from our parents or others who show us compassion. A compassionate attitude toward undesirable aspects or limitations does not mean giving up trying to improve or giving in to unhealthy tendencies—quite the contrary. What compassion does is to stimulate the creative energies, to make healthy changes. One of the statements that many patients make as they improve is how much better they understand now about people suffering from emotional problems. A similar change in attitude is noticeable in loving family members or friends of the patients.

Even couples who have been married for many years may not know each other deeply. The lack of understanding plays a big part in marital conflicts. The judgmental way of looking at people gives the wrong kind of knowledge. Not that one can avoid making certain judgments; approaching compassionately, and then making whatever judgments have to be made, is the loving way.

Fear and pride play a tremendous role in preventing us from self-examination—fear of finding blemishes and shortcomings and the unwillingness to lose our false pride. Some people refuse psychotherapy or spiritual inquiry for the same reason. If the person also happens to be successful, then the resistance is stronger. A successful professional lady was strongly encouraged to get psychotherapy by the man with whom she had fallen in love in a very inappropriate and unrealistic way. She was following him with her characteristic aggressiveness in spite of all his protests. He cared for her well-being and actively encouraged her to get therapy.

She came for therapy a few times showing superficial interest but always defeating and devaluing it quickly. She focused mostly on her rich heritage, big connections, and important positions. She denied any weak points at all. She succeeded in her attempts to prevent any useful self-examination. And besides, she added another feather to her cap of grandiosity by showing that her friend was wrong. Healthy spirituality encourages people to examine themselves, and to be compassionate and patient.

B. Care

According to Milton Mayeroff, caring is helping the other to grow. I prefer the concept of nurturing rather than helping to grow, because nurturing would include caring for somebody who may not grow any further or somebody who may be dying. Exploitation and other forms of destruction are certainly the antithesis of caring.

What we nurture we love. If the mother's love for the infant is stronger than that of the father, it is primarily because she takes so much greater care of the baby than he does. As we see the growth and unfolding of the potentials of the objects of our care, we experience joy. In that process we grow and transcend ourselves and help others to transcend themselves.

In order to nurture, we need to know what is good for the other. One man's meat may indeed be another man's poison. Open and honest communication is important in understanding what is genuinely nurturing. An unselfish attitude enables one to see the other's needs and potentials more objectively. Parents who decide what is good for their children without understanding their genuine potentials are doing them a great disservice.

One of the big mistakes that some people make in choosing their life's companion is using a shopping strategy—buying a finished product that one can continue to use. These people forget the importance of growing up in a relationship. Instead they are disappointed, dismayed, and sometimes desperate when they notice their companion has room to grow. In fact I believe one of the best chances for a deep and lasting relationship is provided by the presence of room for growth on the part of the partners who are willing to nurture each other.

In adversarial types of relationship between couples one partner tries hard to prevent the other from growing. It is not at all uncommon for a spouse to sabotage the therapeutic gains of his or her partner. Even among people who are apparently healthy and well adjusted, elements of such problems are prevalent. A lady physician whom I know very closely told me how surprised her friends and acquaintances of both sexes were when they found out that her husband was helping her a great deal to advance professionally and otherwise.

Care also involves plenty of patience. I learned this as a small child. I used to love garden plants and used to put twigs in the soil to grow new plants. Knowing that the twigs develop roots as they begin to grow and being impatient, I used to pull the twigs out every day to see whether the roots were growing. Several dead twigs later, I learned to be patient and leave the roots alone. That paid off and I learned to wait and watch for new leaves coming out rather than look for the roots.

Nurturing is emphasized by all religions. Healthy spirituality does it well because of its open mind and courage, but sick religiosity tends to manipulate and control the object of nurturing.

C. Respect

Respicere, the root of the word 'respect', means to look at. It involves accepting the other person's individuality. The knowledge of the other person's weaknesses can lead to exploitation unless there is respect and care.

The lowest persons in the social hierarchy suffer not only from economic disadvantage but also from the lowered self-esteem. Jesus, Buddha, Mohammed, and Gandhi took pains to give the sense of acceptance to the persons rejected by society. These great men, unlike radical revolutionaries, did not just turn the tables; they created an atmosphere where all could be accepted.

Respect helps us to let ourselves and others be our genuine selves. Authoritarian and domineering relationships lack respect. The mass manipulators of Huxley's *Brave New World* and Orwell's *1984* are no respectors of persons or of the ideals of love, courage, and wisdom. Fear and respect often get confused. What dictators and authoritarians of various hues instill in others is fear, and not genuine respect. When religious fanatics talk about love of God, they are really speaking of fear, rather than genuine love. When genuine mystics of all religions talk about love of God, they include real respect rather than fear as one of the elements of love.

Because of our respect for those we love, our care is guided by their own direction of growth rather than by our own agenda, hidden or explicit. The former happens with healthy spirituality and the latter with unhealthy religiosity. While bonsai have their own beauty, the same is not true for human beings, whose growth is stunted by excessive controls.

D. Responsibility

Kierkegaard argued that marriage is responsibility and romantic love is irresponsibility. In general, responsibility is equated with duty; that is society's expectation of an individual or a group. The deeper meaning of responsibility is our ability to respond to the needs of others. What is generally expected and what a particular individual needs are not always the same. Respect for the other's individuality and genuine care leads to responding to the other's need authentically.

In many relationships, conflicts arise from a partner's failure to respond to the other's needs. Some partners are so self-centered they are mostly concerned about meeting their own needs and not those of the other person. Similarly, group narcissism and group egoism tends to prevent response to other groups' needs. We are not our brother's keepers, but if we are genuinely brotherly we respond to the needs of our brethren within our own limitations.

Taking responsibility for oneself is an important part of self-affirmation. Those who do not respond to their own needs often become a burden to others who love them. The neurotically self-sacrificing martyrs are really burdening others to meet those needs that they (the 'martyrs') can meet themselves far better and more easily. It is as wasteful as getting somebody else to feed us instead of using our own healthy hands.

II. Deep Love

By deep love, I mean all close relationships. Not just between couples or lovers, but between friends, family members, or any others. It involves an intense degree of the four basic elements of love already discussed. It also involves trust, interdependence, liking, commitment, and shared identity. We will look into these factors in some detail.

A. Trust

Kalidasa, the greatest Sanskrit poet, is famous for his metaphors. One of his most beautiful metaphors is about love: deer scratches the outer corner of its eye against the tip of the stag's horn, so trusting is the relationship between them. Her deep love gives the deer the courage. No cool and rational deer would take such chances; only a passionately loving, deeply trusting deer would do it. Then again, even the deer would learn a dear lesson if it keeps getting hurt.

There is an old saying that where there is no trust there is no love. With openness and trust comes deeper understanding. Trust always involves risk. That is the risk one has to take in order to cross the abyss of one's separateness and reach out to the depth of another from one's own depth. It may seem to be a foolish venture to those who prefer security above everything else.

With trust we let our guards down and show our true selves. It opens us to the possibility of a stronger relationship based on deeper knowledge; it also opens us to the possibility of ridicule and rejection. As the old saying expresses, once bitten, twice shy. Those who have experienced rejection and hurt when they were open and vulnerable may defend against repetition of the bad experience by not trusting, by being defensive.

Basic trust develops in children in the first few years of life if they have fairly consistent and adequate care. As any society becomes increasingly competitive and legalistic, people become less trusting. Children growing up in such an atmosphere risk paranoia. Or they may rebel and go to the opposite extreme of naively trusting without adequate caution. This is not uncommon in my clinical experience.

If we are alienated from ourselves, if we do not let our defenses down and see our own true self, to that extent, we do not trust ourselves. If we do not trust ourselves, we cannot trust others. Then we resort to various defenses to protect ourselves and to control others. Healthy spirituality gives a sense of self-acceptance and courage to be open and vulnerable to trust.

B. Interdependence

Life is a matter of interdependence. In reality there is no self-made man. The closer a relationship, the greater the interdependence. Depending on the relating partners, the give and take may vary tremendously but it is never a totally one-way street. In the relationship between a mother and a young child, the former gives far more but also receives satisfaction and meaning in the process. The child depends on the mother for its life; the mother depends on the child for greater meaning in her life. As the child grows, it responds in its own way and the interdependence goes through many changes.

The problem of too much dependence has been discussed so much that I would say only a few words about it and then I will focus on the equally important but often neglected problem of too much independence. The person who is excessively dependent on others does not use his/her own abilities and skills appropriately. Hence the abilities, skills, and autonomy of such a person stay weak, underdeveloped. Moreover, dependent people are insecure and unhappy, always afraid of losing their support system.

Excessive independence is caused by the fear of dependence, fear of even a healthy level of dependence. Because of the fear of dependence, many people go to the extreme of independence. I have treated many individuals who have this problem. Some of them have become financially and emotionally so independent that they do not care to relate deeply to anybody. It is not hard to see that they are not really happy. All the defenses these individuals put up in order to keep their love needs blocked and repressed give away the secret. Cooperative and creative relationships are interdependent.

The very principle of cooperation is giving and taking, is sharing. Competition, on the other hand, is striving to get the maximum for oneself. The "me generation" finds it hard to share. Sharing the pie is getting only a piece of it; and the larger the number of shares, the smaller the piece. What may be true in economics is not always true in human relationships. *Happiness shared is happiness increased and multiplied; not happiness divided and reduced.* Giving something without good "trade off" is foolish economically; in fact the wise policy is to give something for the maximum profit in return. Not so in human relationships. In human relationships, within certain limits, giving is itself strengthening, invigorating, and beneficial to the giver. It is like healthily exercising one's muscles.

One of Buddha's greatest teachings was about the interdependence of all. And when a Buddhist monk or a Hindu yogi takes alms from others, it is also a symbol of interdependence. In theistic religions God seeks man and, of course, man seeks God. The idea of God becoming man to save humankind (as in Christianity and Hinduism) exemplifies God's interest in us. Unhealthy religiosity promotes heavily authoritarian and hierarchical forms of interdependence of people. Healthy spirituality promotes brotherly/sisterly interdependence.

C. Liking

We hear statements such as "I love you but I don't like you." Although different people might mean different things by such a statement, I believe it is difficult to love intimately without liking. Of course, even in the best of relationships some dislike about some words or actions is bound to happen, but an overall feeling of liking is an integral part of deep love. Love in general, as I described earlier, is quite possible without significant liking. I imagine that is what people basically mean when they say "I love you but I don't like you."

Liking and disliking can depend to an extent on what aspect of the other person one focuses. Sexual turn-on or turn-off can depend to an extent on the focus of attention. One can focus too much on one's own or another person's negative aspect and develop a strong dislike. Similarly, one can focus excessively on only the positive aspect and develop an immoderately strong liking.

Mrs. Strange, wife of an Internist whom I treated several years ago, showed strange ways of liking. This young lady was carrying on an affair with a con-artist who was ugly looking compared to her handsome, well-built husband. Mrs. Strange had no explanation at all for her liking for this 'other man', who had not only used her monetarily and physically, but also given her herpes. She liked him so much that she carried around naked pictures of him in her wallet. She knew he was also carrying on with other women. His flattering words and special attention were enough to twist all her perceptions in his favor, find excuses for his wrongdoings, and like him. Dr. Strange apparently was too busy with his practice to give enough attention to his wife. Moreover, the fun of enjoying forbidden fruit was too enticing for our young lady. She identified more with her lover than her husband.

When a couple's relationship begins to fall apart, the partners sometimes focus on each other's faults and failures. In this process they begin to dislike each other all the more. As that happens, matters get worse. In certain types of relationship, partners stay together although they dislike each other and cause unhappiness.

D. Commitment
Deep love is not a matter of 'falling' accidentally into something like a drunkard falling into a ditch. It involves making choices and an emotional investment. In other words it involves the will. We cannot make one choice without giving up several other choices. Nor can we make an emotional investment without making some important choices. One of the common problems of our times is the making of firm commitments. Influenced by the idea of disposable things and maximum opportunism in the "one life to live," strong commitments appear foolish. One smart bachelor defended his position rather crudely saying "Why keep a cow when there is plenty of milk easily available in the market?" For us busy moderns, commitment seems to be the sacred cow of the past. However, if we want to experience deep love and the joyful fruits thereof, we have no other choice.

When we make a strong commitment, it binds us in one way. At the same time it frees us in many ways. Freedom without boundaries and limitations loses itself and becomes a spent force. As Gandhi observed, in making a vow one is freeing more than binding oneself. Similarly in making a commitment one is gaining more genuine freedom. Religion demands commitment from its members, the beneficial effects of which overflow into other areas. Also the virtues of courage, prudence, and compassion promote commitment. Even fanatic religion fosters commitment.

E. Shared Identity
Shared identity is very important for any deep relationship. When people fall in love, they may overlook the differences in their individual identities and expect their romantic feelings to make their relationship lasting and happy. They are mistaken. Without a deeply shared identity, relationships remain shaky and superficial. Or more commonly the relationship falls apart.

The Bible teaches the couple to leave their parents and become one flesh and one blood. Biological fusion is impossible, even psychological symbiosis is unhealthy. What the Bible obviously intends is for the couple to have an intense shared identity. From being 'you' and 'me', they truly become 'we'. Such intense identity is possible only in deep love although a less intense but broader universal identity is part and parcel of mature spirituality. (More about this in the chapter on Identity.)

Being Lovable

What is often neglected in the literature on love is the importance of being lovable. Love, particularly deep love, cannot flourish—or even sustain for too long—without some response from the other. On our part, therefore, we must not only actively love but also be positively lovable. That means we must let the other person know us, be respectable, communicate our need, accept nurturance, be trustworthy, likeable, interdependent, and willing to share our identity. Without such qualities we will be fending off the other's love. All these characteristics are emphasized by religions. Some people go to an extreme in trying to be lovable and become 'doormats'. Hence the criticism that christianity (and other religions) promotes a slave morality. As one of my patients put it, the people who need a door mat are the ones with dirty shoes. Genuinely lovable people have healthy self-love.

Love and Religion

If religion at its best can be reduced to one word, that would be *love*. Great spiritual masters of all religions preached about the various elements of love and set personal examples of how to love oneself and others. Jesus summed up the Law and the Commandments as love of God and love of fellow human beings. Most radically, Jesus commanded us to love our enemies and to do good to those who hate us.

The Bible declared the importance of love in I John 4:16, "God is love and anyone who lives in love is living with God and God is living in him." Mahabharata teaches: "In joy and sorrow, in pleasure and pain, one should act toward others as one would act toward oneself." This is obviously another expression of the Golden Rule. The essential teaching of Jainism is "ahisma" or nonviolence to all creatures. That means love of all creation.

Buddha taught compassion and interdependence. Matrceta, one of Buddha's followers, described Buddha as a friend with good intentions even toward his enemies. The Enlightened One sought virtue even in those who found fault with him constantly. He taught as much by his good examples as he did by his teachings.

Rabbi Hillel expressed the golden rule by telling people not to do to their fellow creatures what was hateful to themselves. Mosaic Law demands fairness and goodwill to strangers. When he was asked to give a maxim to conduct one's life by, Confucius replied that the answer lies in the word "shu". "Shu" means to love others with the same heart with which we love ourselves.

One of the five pillars of Islam is the duty to practice charity and help the needy. The Koran teaches its followers to repay evil with good, so that by such deeds the enemy will become a friend instead.

Healthy spirituality supports and fosters each one of the elements of love. It promotes open-minded knowledge of oneself and others; it fosters self-respect and respect for everyone else; it inculcates the spirit of nurturing the self and others; it encourages compassion, which involves the active response to the needs of others and oneself. It also helps people to trust, to accept interdependence, to like oneself and fellow beings, to make strong commitments when appropriate, and to have a universal identity. Unhealthy religiosity by its close-mindedness, fears, narcissism, egoism, and narrow identity blocks genuine love. Thereby unhealthy religiosity promotes clannishness and hate of others.

William Johnston points out in *The Inner Eye of Love* that mysticism is the highest aspect of all great religions. And the crowning aspect of mysticism is a universal love—an unrestricted love that extends to all beings including enemies. It involves a deep love of God, but it is not the "pseudo love" of God divorced from love of the world; it is the kind of love that manifests itself in good Samaritans. Johnston makes it clear that unrestricted love does not mean perfect love. It is a love that transcends narrow boundaries and goes on and on, such as Mother Teresa of Calcutta demonstrates. It is the kind of love that brings enlightenment.

In fact, for Johnston, faith is "knowledge born of religious love."[4] He contrasts faith, the infrastructure of religious experience, with belief which is the superstructure. Belief is conditioned by cultural and historical factors. The followers of all the great religions are deeply united in faith although they differ greatly in their beliefs. Obviously, many Christians would disagree with Johnston on this point; for many individuals, faith and belief are one.

Loving the Enemy—There is a widespread notion that it is foolish to try to love one's enemy, that at best one can only tolerate the opponent. Many a self-styled realist pooh-poohs the idea as another sickly creation of idealistic imagination.

I believe loving the enemy is not only practical; it is wise and pragmatic. I do not mean a romantic love nor a deep love but love in general. If we need not have anything to do with the enemy, then a benign indifference or neutrality is fine. But if we have to deal with our enemy for any reason, then a loving approach is indeed the wise one. I will explain this later.

Now, who is the enemy? My dictionary says: "One who is antagonistic." If the one who is antagonistic lives in another part of the country or world and you have nothing really to do with this person, then so be it. But imagine you have to work with the antagonist in the same job. Or imagine you and your spouse got into big conflicts and got a nasty divorce with the help of two bright attorneys who played the adversarial role to the hilt. You hate the guts of your former beloved; you cannot stand the sight of that devilish creature and you will never forget the pain and suffering he/she caused you. At the same time, you have two small children in common. So, in spite of your antagonism, you have to deal with each other. Now, is it wiser to keep the antagonism or to have a loving attitude? Of course, not the deep love you once had but love in general, a basic knowing, respecting, caring, and responding approach.

What is true for individuals is true for groups. If one group need not have anything to do with an antagonistic group, then indifference and distance work fine. Which is not the case between neighboring countries and various groups that are interdependent. Marx's class war is indeed a hateful solution. The superpowers are the most powerful antagonists of our time. The future of the human race and of life on earth is in their hands. Therefore, the United States and the Soviet Union have enormous responsibility to have a "loving" relationship.

The basic elements of love—knowledge, care, respect, and responsibility—are possible in dealing with an enemy. The elements of deep love such as an intense level of the above factors, liking, trust, interdependence and commitment, are possible with enemies only to a limited extent. We may not like our enemies at all. That almost goes without saying. We cannot trust them much and become excessively vulnerable to them. We try to keep our interdependence with antagonists to a bare minimum, just enough to serve the common purpose. As far as commitment is concerned, we can try to keep the commitments we make, but we naturally try to avoid making commitments to adversaries over and above what is needed.

There are many reasons why the basic elements of love are extremely important in dealing with enemies. Knowledge of the enemy—true knowledge of both strength and weakness—makes our defenses realistic, neither exaggerated nor inadequate. We create a monstrous picture of the enemies by exaggerating all their bad aspects, overlooking all their good qualities and reading into them our own fantasized fears. I call this 'monsterizing'. Then we fight this imaginary monster and waste our energies and destroy ourselves and the other to a greater or less extent.

A basically respecting and caring attitude keeps our own destructive tendencies down, and keeps our constructive energies flowing. Love does beget love, although not in equal measure and not always from the object of our giving.There is a Sufi saying that love is like an echo; the sound comes back from somewhere. Caring, even caring for pets, has been proven to be therapeutic. Hostile feelingss have been shown to be injurious to our health and well being. This has been clearly demonstrated in stress disorders.

Responding to the genuine and important needs of our enemies reduces tensions and paves the way for better relationships. It has been said that a friend in need is a friend indeed. We can also say that an enemy who responds to our deep need is indeed someone we cannot easily hurt. Gratitude is a universal phenomenon among human beings and animals. Of course, universal doesn't mean always. In fact, Dostoevsky's observation of man as the most ungrateful animal also proves true at times. Yet the odds are certainly in favor of responding to the deep and genuine need of the adversary. At worst, what do we lose by it? What we really lose is any sadistic pleasure in the suffering of another. We may feel superior that we do not have the kind of problem our adversary is having. That is sick pride.

Confucius disagreed with the Mohists' (another Chinese school of thought) advocacy of loving everyone equally. Instead of loving the enemy, he advised to do justice to the enemy. By love Confucius meant deep love. We tend to be unjust to those we hate. In order to do justice, we need to have a modicum of love. In fact, Paul Tillich emphasized that there is no justice without love. Therefore Confucius' teaching to do justice to the enemy is consistent with the idea of loving rather than hating the foe, although this love is not the deep love one has towards friends and family. Religion puts its best foot forward when it actively promotes love, including love of the enemy.

8. ANGER, HATE AND INDIFFERENCE

"Hatred paralyzes life; love releases it. Hatred confuses life; love harmonizes it. Hatred darkens life; love illumines it.' '

> Martin Luther King, Jr.
> (Strength to Love)

"The daily news tells us again and again that, with all his knowledge and with all his refined ways, modern man remains the wildest animal.' '

> Isaac Bashevis Singer
> (U.S. News & World Report, 1983)

"When you visualized a man or a woman carefully, you could always begin to feel pity . . . when you saw the lines at the corners of the eyes, the shape of the mouth, how the hair grew, it was impossible to hate. Hate was just a failure of imagination.' '

> Graham Greene
> (The Power and the Glory)

In order to appreciate the day fully, we need to experience the night. In order to understand the dynamics of love fully, we need to understand the dynamics of hate. Moreover, hate is an extremely important aspect of life in its own right.

Love and hate have been considered as opposites by most people. However, there are some who consider indifference as the real opposite of love. Does it make sense psychologically? Those who claim indifference as the opposite of love argue that when we hate someone we acknowledge the personhood of the other but when we are indifferent to somebody we dehumanize the other, treating the other as a thing. It sounds plausible but it is a shallow argument.

There are three kinds of indifference:

1. Benign indifference—true indifference because of practical limitations.
2. Benevolent indifference that masks love.
3. Indifference that masks hate—malignant indifference.

1. *Benign indifference*—As human beings we have various limitations in spite of our wishes and ideals. If we are facing a crisis, then our attention may be so focused on the crisis that we may overlook the needs or sufferings of others. A man almost drowning in deep waters may be indifferent to another person in the same plight. There are particularly courageous individuals who forget their own need and take care of others even in such situations. Most people may react indifferently to a calamity in a far corner of the world with which they have no connections. All these people are not hateful or noncaring individuals. It is a matter of living within our limited resources.

2. *Benevolent indifference*—As a clinician I come across this rather frequently. Family members of alcohol and drug abusers, after repeated attempts to bail them out of trouble, realize the futility of such an approach. Then the family members are likely to show indifference to the sufferings of the substance abuser. That indifference is born out of the realization that substance abusers benefit by being forced to face their problem. So long as others take care of complications arising from substance abuse, why should the abuser bother to change? Similarly, parents of teenagers with behavior problems learn to stop rescuing them.

In relationships where the partners have too many differences, indifference may be a way to maintain the relationship. I know a good Catholic lady who is broad minded, out-going, charitable, and loving. Her husband is dependent, reserved, introverted, and rather a fanatic in his religious life. Her marriage is not happy, but because of her religious faith and her concern for her husband she does not want to divorce him. When she attempted to have a more intense and intimate relationship with him, it caused much conflict. Then she learned to cope with the situation by a sort of indifference. This approach has worked much better. I know of many such relationships.

3. *Malignant indifference*—By this I mean indifference that masks hate. This leads to dehumanization of the other as part of the hating process. The hate underlying such indifference shows up in subtle and sometimes not so subtle ways. The persons with malignant indifference may show signs of relief or even rejoicing at the sufferings of the people they secretly hate. I am reminded of a Christian lady who was apparently being indifferent about her ex-

husband whom she had divorced after years of marital conflict. Then she heard from a female friend that her ex-husband was miserable after a failed love relationship. Our nice lady gathered a lot of information about her former husband's unsuccessful love and all his misery. As she talked about it, her face lit up. She had a twinkle in her eyes and a cheerful smle. It was very clear that she hated her ex-husband. However, she denied any hatred for him, saying that she, being a good Christian, had only love for him. However, when her apparent rejoicing at his misery was pointed out, she was first offended. Later, she did reflect on it and admitted she did have a lot of hate. Subsequently she worked on the hate and overcame it. As she became more genuinely loving, she dropped her good Christian mask.

It is clear from the above discussion that indifference (that is, true indifference) is not the opposite of love. Hate is really the opposite of love and it will become abundantly clear as we look at the various aspects of hate. But first we will examine the difference between anger and hate.

Anger and Hate:

There is often much confusion regarding anger and hate. Aristotle's discussion of anger and hate in his *Rhetoric*, Book II, is highly relevant for us in this chapter. His ideas are as follows: Anger results from an offense against us. Hatred may occur even without any offense. For example, we may hate somebody for what we perceive as his or her bad character. Anger is aimed at returning pain to the offender; hate aims at doing harm to its object. Anger is directed at individuals whereas hate may be directed against classes of people. (We may modify this idea and say anger is more focused but hatred may be diffuse.) Whereas anger has accompanying pain, hatred does not. The angry individual can pity his/her offender but the hater does not pity his/her objects of hate. The hater wishes the annihilation of his or her enemies. The angry individual is satisfied by the suffering of the offenders. While time cures anger, hate stays on. These psychological insights of Aristotle are so good that they are not easy to improve upon.

Fear (realistic fear) and anger are healthy emotions. They help to protect and preserve ourselves and our self-esteem. Hatred, on the other hand, is destructive to us and to others. We have already seen the way caution helps. Similarly anger alerts us about an injury to our self or our own self-esteem that has already occurred.

Human aggression may result from anger and realistic fear, or from hate. This is a very important distinction. To consider all aggression as bad is totally unrealistic. Erich Fromm's ideas about benign aggression versus malignant aggression (in *The Anatomy of*

Human Destructiveness) are of tremendous help in understanding this point.

As Fromm demonstrated, benign aggression is a response to the vital interests of an organism; it is adaptive and biologically programmed; it is reactive to a threat. Animals and man show benign aggression. However, man alone shows malignant aggression, cruelty, and destructiveness that are not basically adaptive. One only needs to recapture the negative highlights of human history to prove the point.

In *Human Aggression,* Anthony Storr points out that normal aggression turns to hatred when there is an admixture of revenge with the aggression. He further notes that the tendency to hurt those who are already defeated or those who are really weaker is motivated by the spirit of vengeance. In everyday life, when we "take it out" on someone, as the phrase goes, we are crossing the boundary of anger and entering the territory of hatred. The *it* that we are taking out on the other is not anger but hate, as Storr emphasizes.

In my clinical experience those who were abused as children (and therefore grew up experiencing hatred) tend to react with varying degrees of hatred in situations where others would only react with a mild or moderate degree of anger. Some of them would take it out on their spouses or children. Some others would pout and give the silent treatment for several days for small infringement. One of my patients who was abused as a child, got into a big fight with her husband once for forgetting to deposit one check in the bank, although his forgetfulness that time was not going to cause any major problems. The only inconvenience she had from his forgetting was that she had to go and deposit the check in the bank and balance the checkbook. She fought with him for a week over it. Their marriage has been stormy all along because of similar conflicts.

Those who experience hatred rather than love in the formative years of their lives tend to sense threat and humiliation in situations where no real reasons for such perceptions exist. In other situations there may be true reason for a mild level of fear or anger, but instead these people react with hate. Hate indeed begets hate. Hate experienced in childhood leaves the individual prone to become hateful. Of course corrective experience and therapy can relieve the tendency to hate. However, corrective experiences and therapy become difficult for these individuals because of their tendency to perceive rejection and hate in the attitudes and actions of others, including therapists.

If anger is allowed to accumulate and linger, it can very well turn into hatred. Therefore, when certain religious denominations denounce anger, they are only setting the stage for the growth of hatred, as we saw in the case of Jane in Chapter Five. It is far better to be aware of the anger and deal with it. Talking it over with the person who caused it may be the best approach. However, talking about it with someone who is understanding or by expressing the anger in actions such as punching a punching bag may be the best approach at other times. If the anger is about something unimportant, often one can just let it go. The Biblical teaching not to let the sun go down on one's anger makes excellent sense.

Characteristics of Hate
    In general, opposites of the various elements of love can be seen in hate.
    A. *Ignorance and Illusion*—This is the most basic factor in hate. A good example is what Jerome Frank calls "the image of the enemy." The image of the enemy is made up of all kinds of negative impressions, judgments, and distortion of facts and figures about the enemy. Everything we dislike, depreciate, and find deplorable easily becomes part of that image. The enemy is seen as barbaric, sadistic, unscrupulous, greedy, venomous, brutal, seductive, and the like. Our selective perception makes it easy for us to overlook the positive attributes of the enemy and focus just on the negative aspects. Even when we are confronted by a good quality of the enemy, we explain it away by saying "Yes, but it is really just a ploy or propaganda."
    Frank gives examples from international relationships that show the way the image of the enemy works. Public opinion polls in 1942 and 1966 in the U. S. showed an interesting shift. Germans and Japanese were considered cruel, treacherous, and warlike in 1942 but not in 1966. Bad characteristics were attributed to Russians in 1966 and good features were attributed to Japanese and Germans.[1]
    A former colleague of mine saw various international issues basically in terms of democracy versus communism. He was more widely read and traveled than many of my colleagues. However, his tendency to fit various political, economic, cultural, and religious issues into the format of democracy versus communism led him to have some interestingly distorted views. For example, he viewed India as a non-democratic country because India is a non-aligned country and has a friendly relationship with the Soviet Union as well as the U. S. When I asked him about the definition of democracy as the "government of the people, by the people, and for the people," he said that it doesn't matter. At one point he said even if India is considered a democracy by a lot of people, it is not a "real democracy." By real democracy he meant anti-Moscow and pro-Washington.
    His argument about "real democracy" reminded me of an interesting experience I had while working in Jamaica. A foreign tourist spontaneously asked me "how much is it in 'real money'?"

when I told him about my fees in Jamaican dollars. Misinterpretation of differences is often at the root of prejudice. Anything strange or foreign to one's own appearance or outlook can be the focus of such misinterpretation. The words foe and foreign are synonymous in Latin. In Japanese the word for different and the word for wrong are the same. Misinterpretation of the action of the one we hate maintains the process of hate and prevents the forces of love from working. Anyone who genuinely tries to intervene and point out to the enemies the fallacy of their understanding of each other finds it very frustrating. Let me give one of my own sad personal experiences to illustrate this point.

I have been very close to two brothers for many years. They were loving siblings in the early years. Gradually they grew apart, particularly after they got married. Then they became bitter enemies, mostly over financial matters. If I say anything good about the one, the other gets angry with me. When the older brother gave considerable support for the orphanage, the other sibling interpreted the action as a way of relieving guilt over illegitimate children. Even the special caring that the young brother showed to his own children was misinterpreted by the older sibling as plain sick pride. As far as I know, the only thing they both have against me is that I am friendly to the other. To top everything off, they are both religious people, one more so than the other.

Diogenes (around 350 B.C.) noted the interesting way people interpret differences. This man of wisdom observed that, if somebody used his/her middle finger instead of the index finger for pointing, that person would be considered mad. That boils down to an individual being only a finger's breadth away from being judged crazy. What a mad world!

Mental pictures of the out-groups are characterized by negative impressions. Almost always there is some grain of truth somewhere in the mass of falsehood that makes up the negative image. This is true in self-hate also. The little grain of truth only makes the process of denial strong. Whenever the person is confronted by the falsity of his/her hateful impressions, the person holds up the small grain of truth to refute the genuine overall truth. In the process of hate, misperceptions are defended carefully. Keeping physical and psychological distances are common ways of preserving prejudice. Even as gentle and great a soul as Charles Lamb is reported to have had a strong dislike for somebody. And Mr. Lamb preserved this dislike by never even meeting the enemy.

In the process of hate, empathy and compassion are blocked off. In *Compassion and Self-Hate* psychoanalyst Theodore Rubin observes that compassion is the best antidote for self-hate and hate of others. Graham Greene's contention that hate is the failure of imagination contains a great truth. In hate the imagination is partial; it is used selectively to focus on the negative aspects and to block off the positive aspects. The process of blocking empathy and compassion leads to hardening of the heart and further closure of the mind. And that easily leads to dehumanization. Dehumanization is an easy way out of the humane feelings toward other individuals. One of the most effective techniques used in the training of torturers is the dehumanization of victims. By viewing the enemy as some kind of bad abstraction, it becomes easy to be cruel to them. The enemy becomes targets to be eliminated. What is often not recognized is that the dehumanizer is alienating himself/herself from his/her true human self also in the process. Modern technology has skyrocketed dehumanization. Eliminating a target by remote control is worlds apart from facing the enemy in hand-to-hand combat.

There is also the tendency to dichotomize everything into good and evil or right and wrong. Grey areas are forcibly put into black or white categories. An American President characterized the nonaligned movement as immoral. The Biblical idea of "he who is not with me is against me" can cause unnecessary trouble when applied indiscriminately.

Psychiatrist Charles Pinderhughes has an interesting hypothesis about "differential bonding." He bases his hypothesis on ethological, biological, and psychological studies which have shown attachment or bonding behavior toward some objects and aggressive or avoidant behavior toward other objects. Lorenz's studies on birds and fish, Harlow's studies on monkeys, and Bowlby's studies on humans are prominent examples. One of the most important hypotheses put forward by Pinderhughes is: "The object of the affiliative-affectionate linkage is aggrandized and the object of the differentiative-aggressive linkage is renounced."[2] These processes produce false beliefs based on projections.

With such a process, irrational interconnections of a chain of negative impressions can occur. For example a patient of mine once told me how he lost respect for Reverend Jerry Falwell because Falwell invited Senator Edward Kennedy to speak at Falwell's church. According to my patient, Kennedy is a social-welfare supporter and therefore a socialist which really means a communist. And any preacher who invites a Godless communist to his church is bad news. Interestingly this patient is a macho man who abuses and exploits his wife, and is obviously more fundamentalistic a Christian than Falwell.

Dislike—We like what is in accordance to our taste, what enhances our self-esteem, or protects our self. On the contrary, we dislike what is opposed to our taste, our sense of security, or our self-esteem. We dislike people who bring up bad memories or threaten our well being; we dislike bearers of bad news. We dislike everything that interferes with our cherished identity. There is a saying in India that one finds fault with everything done by the woman one dislikes. We see the actions of the people we dislike in a highly unfavorable light. This leads to further escalation of hate. In the absence of an empathic and compassionate outlook, the dislike continues. Dislike and selective perception of negative aspects of oneself or others lead to contempt.

Contempt—In admiration we look up to somebody; in worship (or more aptly, "worshup", as per Mathew Fox) we look even further up. But in hate we look down. We view with contempt the person or the group that we hate. If we are hard-pressed to admit something good about the enemy, it is drowned out in the overall negative outlook. With contempt comes rejection.

Religion often plays a significant role in the victimizer's contempt for the victims. For Christian colonialists, the heathen subjects were a condemned lot; for exploiting whites, the blacks had no souls; for macho men, the women were weak characters and temptresses. Excessive guilt produced by unhealthy religiosity causes self-contempt. Those who are contemptuous of others often show exclusive identity.

Exclusive Identity—Hate and exclusive identity go hand in hand. Even in self-hate one part of us (the ideal self) has a proud and exclusive identity that rejects one's own real self. When the caste system was strong in India, the upperclass Hindus excluded the lowest class of untouchables from their Hindu identity. The attitude of exclusive identity led to hateful behaviors toward the untouchables by the high caste Hindus. As we exclude somebody from our identity it becomes easy to condemn, exploit, and destroy that person. What is close to our identity is dear to us and we are protective of it. I suspect that is one reason for some Christian fundamentalists' support of the racist white government in South Africa.

Not responding to other's needs—Even when we have the ability and the resources to respond to the needs of our perceived enemy, we refrain from doing so. Moreover, in the process of hate, we rejoice at the sufferings of our enemies, one of which is their inability to meet their needs. Sadism is part of hate and cruelty. Nothing is so satisfying to sadistic tendency as the sights and sounds of the suffering of others. Political and military leaders have a way of pretending, at least at times, as though other countries don't have the need for security from external threats and stability in internal conditions. "We are the good guys; they can just trust that we have no evil intent; everything we do is totally for defensive purposes" is their attitude. The same people refuse to take the same attitude when the role is reversed.

Couples with marital conflicts frequently keep making the partner's needs worse by various manipulations. One young couple was escalating their conflicts for a few months. The husband has a strong need for attention and the wife has a strong need for security. The man was making the woman's need for security worse by his unpredictable temper and his criticism of her. The woman was making his need for attention worse by putting more energy into work. They were willing to look at the problem and make changes, unlike many others who go on with the proces of hate.

Opportunism and Exploitation—While we show commitment to our friends, we show opportunism and exploitation towards our enemies. We try to enhance the power and glory of our self or our group at the expense of our enemies whenever we get a chance. That serves the twin purpose of self-aggrandisement and weakening of the enemy. "Strike when the iron is hot" goes the old saying. Here again, unlike the very limited extent of such behavior in animals, man has used all his intelligence to broaden these evil tendencies. Probably the worst racial oppression and exploitation has occurred where Puritan Calvinistic ethics prevailed, such as in South Africa.

Hostile independence—The phrase hostile independence is used here to denote our tendency to be the least dependent on our enemies. This tendency can extend to all areas of relationships. It is all the more strong in those areas where we feel we could be most vulnerable to our enemies. Interdependence, common interests, and common obligations are important in any loving relationship. In hate the opposite tendencies prevail. The unfortunate consequence is that the opportunities for moving to a less hateful, more loving relationship are lost. One can even note in different families and other groups the continuation of hate from one generation to the next. For the past few months I have been treating a couple who hate each other, but who are too insecure to go their separate ways. Both of them try hard to be independent of each other—not giving a chance for the other to show kindness or interest.

Mistrust—Trust, as we saw in the section on Love, involves being vulnerable to hurt. By not trusting our enemies we are protecting ourselves from harm. By taking a step further and positively mistrusting them and keeping constant vigilance for malice on their part, we keep the process of hate in high gear. Authoritarian and insecure leaders like Jim Jones show clear evidence of such tendencies. For one thing, they try to control their own group tightly; for another, they escalate tension several-fold by constant vigilance and misinterpretation of every possible move of outsiders.

Destructiveness—As surely as we want to nurture what we love, so clearly do we want to destroy what we hate. Love is the constructive force of sentient beings; hate is the destructive force in human beings. Benign aggression from anger or from fear of a real threat is part of our normal survival instinct. By destroying our enemy, we feel safe and powerful. It adds to our pride and security. With more pride and less caution, the destructiveness worsens.

In the Biblical account of history, the first instance of human death was not a natural death but a murder, that of brother killing brother. Along the lines of Isaac Singer's observation one can say that modern man remains worse than the wildest animals in some ways. Wild animals kill for survival, not out of hate.

Religion and Hate

"Whosoever hateth his brother is a murderer: and ye know that no murderer hath eternal life abiding in him." I John 3:15. The healthy side of religion promotes love and prevents hate. One of the functions of the golden rule is to prevent hate. Buddha taught that only love can overcome hate. Similar views can be found in various religions and the teachings of thinkers like Baruch Spinoza. Counter hatred only adds more fuel to the fire of hatred. Mahatma Gandhi and Martin Luther King, Jr. showed how to apply this principle in a socio-political context. Thomas Merton (in *New Seeds of Contemplation*) views hell as hatred and sinners as people who hate.

As we saw in Chapter 3, the spiritually mature person is a true peacemaker who works through understanding and negotiations, thereby minimizing possibilities for tension and hatred. In his famous letter from the Birmingham jail, King outlined the four basic steps of a nonviolent campaign: "(1) Collection of the facts to determine whether injustices are alive; (2) Negotiations; (3) Self-purification; and (4) Direct action."[3] And the direct actions were peaceful protests and noncooperation (such as civil disobedience).

However, the fanatical side of religion is one of the most potent sources of hate. It is interesting to look into the manner in which religious fanaticism creates and fosters hate through every element of hate we have examined.

Religious fanaticism promotes ignorance and illusion by limiting knowledge. It also causes dichotomous thinking—seeing everything in black and white terms. Other people's beliefs and religious practices are easily misinterpreted. Critical thinking, doubts, and questions are discouraged. People are made scared of God's wrath if they dare to think differently. Other religions and world views are seen as evil.

Religious fanatics have intense dislike for other religions and world views. Whatever is done by other religious groups is seen through dark glasses. Even the obviously good deeds done by other religious groups are explained away as basically unimportant or as filled with evil intent. Fanatics show contempt for outsiders. Others are seen as children of darkness, Satan's followers, devil's disciples, and the like. For Ayatolla Khomeini, America is the land of Satan. Christian fundamentalist Billy Sunday's patriotic sermons included statements such as, "If you turn Hell upside down, you would find 'Made In Germany' on the bottom." There is a sense of keeping one's own purity by rejecting others.

Exclusive identity is an obvious feature of religious fanaticism. The fanatic Christian considers his/her group as the only true Christians. The fanatic Moslem does the same and so on. The negative identity of "I am not a heathen, or I am not a Jew, or I am not a Hindu," or whatever group one hates, may be even more important than the positive identification of oneself with the depth of one's own faith. An evangelist declared that all humans are *not* children of God; only his brand of Christians are children of God. Others are just children of Adam. Another electronics evangelist who opposes any close relationship with the Soviet Union claims that the lamb and the lion would lie together only when the former is inside the stomach of the latter.

Religious fanatics are masters of the art of not responding to the needs of others. They do not see the significance of the sense of security and self-esteem for everyone. In fact, they do enjoy threatening the security and self-esteem of others. Humiliating and scaring them are common techniques fanatics use in converting others.

Opportunism and exploitation are often practiced by religious fanatics. Any opportunity to enlarge the group's size or power is not only good for the group here on earth, but it also brings more blessing from heaven. Exploitation of young minds is cleverly conducted by many religious cults. A mixture of fear and guilt, followed by a strong dose of hope hereafter, and a deep sense of belonging in a group here are time-tested religious formulas to gain new members.

Hostile independence—'separatism' or keeping away from the 'evil world'—is also clearly seen in religious fanaticism. In trying to be pure, unpolluted, and saintly, fanatics keep away from others whom they consider spiritually sick. Even some 'Christian psychiatrists' tell their good Christian clients to remain most intimate with their own kind. Often the only reason offered to approach other groups is to convert them, to augment the power of one's own group.

Distrust and destructiveness are also essential features of unhealthy religiosity. History is marred by Holy Wars of various magnitudes. Besides such gross instances, there are plenty of examples of destructiveness in community, family, and individual levels. Although extremely rare, human sacrifices still happen in India. In 1982, a member of a Christian fundamentalist group in West Virginia paddled his 23-month-old son for several hours leading to the boy's death. I have treated several individuals whose fanatically religious parents were child abusers. Some of these cases were daughters of fundamentalist ministers who were sexually abused by their fathers.

Particularly ironic and tragic are the ways in which prayers and peace-promoting ideas are converted to destructive means. In 1982 Bob Jones, Jr. (the Chancellor of Bob Jones University), angered by then-Secretary of State Alexander Haig's refusal to issue a visa to Irish Protestant extremist Ian Paisley, prayed that God "destroy him [Haig] quickly and utterly." In April 1986, a Hindu swami gave a new twist to an old pacifist couplet: "shower flowers on the enemy who pricks you with a thorn." The swami's version: "He who pricks you with a thorn, pierce him with a spear in return and teach him an unforgettable lesson."

Referring to how people have justified and glorified exploitation of others in the name of God, Sam Keen notes: "It was he [God] who gave America a "manifest destiny," granted Britain the dignity of bearing "the white man's burden," allowed the Japanese to create a greater East-Asia Co-prosperity sphere, helped Mussolini to rebuild the glorious Roman Empire, and prompted Hitler to envision the thousand year Reich."[4]

Holy Wars are particularly vicious and prolonged. Participants in Holy Wars do not have the restraints of conscience since the religious cause takes care of any sense of guilt. The hope of instant salvation or even a special place in heaven and high honor on earth makes killing for one's religion extremely attractive. The suicide squads of the Islamic Jihad are among recent examples of this phenomenon. Into such glorious projects, fanatics can pour out their hearts and souls.

Moreover, in being cruel to their enemies, religious fanatics are punishing God's enemies, sort of doing the dirty work for God. In that sense fanatics feel special to the Almighty, in much the same way that the henchmen of kings and dictators feel about their masters. Furthermore, as Jerome Frank observed, Holy Wars have no natural end-points like other wars. Most wars are about control of territory or power over others but in Holy Wars the struggle can go on until the other side is converted or destroyed. Often the fight goes on until both sides are exhausted.[5]

Grace Halsell speculates that a world-wide war might erupt if a group of Jewish fanatics—with support from some Christian Fundamentalists—succeed in their plan to destroy Islam's most holy shrine in Jerusalem.[6] Wouldn't it be the ultimate irony of the destructiveness of religion which preaches love and peace.

All in all, Holy Wars are among the most unholy of human interactions. Only the strong psychological dynamics of hate can drag people down to such depths of degradation and destructiveness. It shows religion at one of its worst.

9. KNOWLEDGE, IGNORANCE, AND WISDOM

"Why do you not of yourselves judge what is right?"

— Luke 12:57

"Believe only what you yourself judge to be true."

— Buddha

"He who knows himself knows others."

— Chinese Proverb

Our capacity to know, ability to think, power of reasoning, and depth of awareness—these set us apart from everything else in the world, and possibly in the universe. In this chapter we will examine several important issues related to knowledge and ignorance and their place in the healthy and unhealthy dynamics of religion.

In the beautiful words of Pascal, "Man is the weakest reed in creation but a thinking reed." We have a tremendous urge to use this capacity to think, a strong thirst for knowledge, a great need to search for truth. That is what has led to human progress. The marvels of scientific and philosophical knowledge and the wonderful products of technology bear witness to this.

At the same time we are pulled from the opposite direction. That is, we also have a strong tendency to play games with our knowledge, awareness, and thinking. That unfortunate tendency—the tendency to lie—is at the root of our problems. This tendency exists because, as T. S. Eliot noted with brilliant poetic insight, we cannot bear very much reality; for it upsets our pride and security. We tend to manipulate and toy with information and awareness that threatens our sense of security or our self-esteem.

With the keen perception of a mystic, Martin Buber asserted (in *Good and Evil*) that the particular evil that human beings introduced into the world is the lie. Furthermore, he noted that this lie is quite different from any little deceits the animals may show from time to time. And the lie is used not just in relationship with others but also in one's relationship to oneself.

These two opposing forces in us—the tendency to know and the tendency to ignore—play a pivotal role in anyone's religious life. The same is true of the group dynamics of religion. "To be or not to be," Hamlet informed us, is the ultimate question. An equally important question is to know or not to know.

Knowledge—Science, philosophy, and religion are different fields in which human beings search for truth. All these emphasize truth. Both in the East and in the West, both in times past and in our own days, the importance of knowledge is recognized.

The widom of the Greeks as expressed in the Delphic motto taught: "Know thyself." Socrates said, "Knowledge is virtue." Similarly the Hindu Vedas (veda means knowledge) advised: "Know yourself", (*Atmanam viddhi* in Sanskrit). All great religious teachers agree on the ultimate importance of the right knowledge. Buddha, for example, taught right knowledge and right mindfulness as two steps in the eightfold path of spiritual growth. The statement of Jesus that the truth shall make us free is well known. The first thing that Jews pray everyday—in fact three times a day—is for knowledge: "Oh grant us knowledge, understanding, insight." Being aware, being truly awake, or being enlightened is particularly emphasized by all religions.

In fact, many religious teachings and practices are meant to increase our awareness of the depth of our being, and alert us to the proper ways to live so that we can fully actualize our potentials. The reading of scriptures and other religious writings is intended for this purpose. Meditation, yoga, fasting, and various religious rituals are ultimately for the same purpose. And the proof of the pudding is in the eating. Awareness without accompanying action is worthless. Faith without works is dead, as the Bible teaches.

Healthy spirituality relies heavily on increasing awareness—raising consciousness if you will—and transforming the individual for the better. Gandhi considered his life a search for Truth, "Experiments with Truth" as the title of his autobiography states. The history of religions is filled with examples of how religious founders and reformers, prophets and mystics, brought about healthy changes in the attitudes and actions of their followers by new awareness.

The physical sciences have increased our knowledge of the physical world, and its application has increased our life span and our creature comforts. Behavioral and social sciences have vastly increased our understanding of how individuals and societies function. Healthy spirituality not only supports these advancements but also tries to spread the benefits of scientific progress. Educational institutions run by religious groups, particularly Christians, have helped greatly to spread knowledge throughout the world. The gurus of ancient India and the teachers of ancient China provided their students not just religious training but an overall education. It is remarkable how psychologically insightful the great spiritual teachers were. Various schools of psychotherapy emphasize insight as a therapeutic goal. And this insight is not an intellectual knowledge but an experiential understanding that leads to healthy change. Behavior therapists do not conceptualize in this way; they help to overcome maladaptive behavior by teaching adaptive behavior. Therefore, behavioral therapy in our sense also involves insight. Cognitive therapists tend to analyze faulty ways of thinking and correct them, thereby solving problems. Similar approaches have been part of healthy religious practices.

Interestingly, in the authoritative book *Theories of Personality* by Hall and Lindsey there is a chapter on Eastern psychology which is in fact a part of Eastern religion. While some cognitive therapists go around as if they are the first ones to discover the problems of faulty thinking, those familiar with Buddhist teachings remember with a smile the opening sentence of Dhammapada, a Buddhist scripture: "All that we are is a result of what we have thought."

Dr. Steven Brena, a pioneer in the treatment of chronic pain, in his book *Yoga and Medicine* describes how yoga, by its holistic approach, enhances the total functioning of a person by enhancing sensory, autonomic, and hormonal (endocrine) systems as well as spirituality.

"The 'Royal Way of Yoga' takes man as he is, with all his handicaps, and brings him above boundaries of material forces to Cosmic Consciousness. . . Along the way, while seeking spiritual realization, man can also discover the key to health, joy, and inner freedom."[1]

The benefits of Meditation are now recognized in psychiatry. In an important article in *The American Journal of Psychiatry*, January 1985, the authors recommended the addition of meditative techniques to psychotherapy. Psychiatry has come a long way from Freud's interpretation of the meditative experience of "oceanic feeling" as a reaction formation of omnipotence to compensate infantile helplessness.

Religion has recognized the importance of science. A Catholic priest and paleontologist, Teilhard de Chardin, a strong proponent of evolution, was an important influence in the Vatican II movement of the Catholic Church which broadened and liberated the church. Baha Ulla, founder of the relatively new Bahai faith, told his followers to follow science if there is conflict between science and religion. What has been said so far may indicate that religion is completely in favor of knowledge, search for truth, and openmindedness. While this is quite true about the healthy side of religion, the opposite holds true for the unhealthy, fanatical side of religion.

Ignorance—In spite of the general importance given to knowledge, one often hears statements such as "ignorance is bliss" or "what you don't know won't hurt you." There is a humorous story recorded in the Hindu epic Mahabharata that illustrates this point:

A great sage named Vibhandaka who lived a saintly life in a forest once happened to see a beautiful woman bathing in a river. He lost control of his sexual desire and had intercourse with a deer. From that union was born a boy who was named Rishyasringa. Vibhandaka decided to make sure his son wouldn't have problems with sexuality. He brought up the son with no contacts at all with women. When Rishyasringa became a young man, it happened that in the local kingdom of Anga there was a drought. According to a prophecy, there would be rain if Rishyasringa could be brought to the country from his forest dwelling.

The most charming courtesans of the kingdom were sent to accomplish this task. A young attractive courtesan approached Rishyasringa when his father was away. Rishyasringa, who had never seen any woman in his life, completely mistook the courtesan for another great ascetic. He interpreted all her feminine features to be the result of years of spiritual exercise. After exchanging greetings, offering him sweets and embracing him a few times as though in salutation, the courtesan left. Rishyasringa had a new experience of ecstasy and a new joy unlike all his previous spiritual highs. When his son told Vibhandaka about the visit from another ascetic, the latter warned him of witches and evil consequences. However, the following day when the father was gone and the courtesan returned, Rishyasringa welcomed her. This time Rishyasringa went off with her, still thinking that she was a sage like himself.

Things worked out well for him because the kingdom got rain and a grateful king gave his own daughter in marriage to Rishyasringa. However, the moral of the story is that keeping someone ignorant to prevent him or her from doing wrong only backfires. Incidentally, those who are opposed to sex education have a great predecessor in Vibhandaka.

Ignorance is usually understood as lack of information. There is another form of ignorance too—ignoring the information already present. The latter type of ignorance may arise because of fear of new ideas or because of prideful attachment to previous ideas.

Unhealthy religiosity favors ignorance apart from the specific information that is approved by the group's authority figure. The group's own ideology is repeatedly emphasized. Other ideas are either prohibited or distorted so that people would easily reject these ideas. Moreover, even contacts with people who might give a different view are restricted by the teachings of fanatical religionists. Various cults are good examples of these. In many cults the newcomers are given false information and unrealistic images   of the cult. People who are already deeply involved with the cult are used to influence the newcomer. The "moonies" tell lies to newcomers, which they call "heavenly deception." Another cult, Children of God, uses what some people call "flirty fishing" —sexual seduction—to attract new members.

All fanatical groups inculcate in their members a strong fear about looking at life from any perspective that is really different from the group's own. Even the Christian psychiatrists warn the committed Christians against outside influences.

Closely allied to ignorance is illusion. While religion is supposed to shatter our ignorance and illusion, especially about the ultimate meaning of life, unhealthy religion creates its own illusions or reinforces other illusions. Religious fanatics play gods, glorifying themselves and condemning others, in the name of their faith. The cult leaders are often minigods and God for them is the ultimate cult leader. The glorification of oneself extends from the narcissistic leader to his favorites. I remember a television evangelist once declaring to his audience that a book written by his wife is the greatest book next to the Bible.

Along with an illusion of one's own narcissistic glory goes the illusion of the evil of others just because they have a different belief. Whether someone is loving, honest, prudent, and courageous does not count. What counts is whether someone belongs to the right group, whether he/she uses the lingo of that group.

There are various illusions connected with religion—illusions of invulnerability, magical power, infallibility, of being above ethical laws and moral consequences and the illusion of wisdom without using reason and doubt.

One of the worst illusions is that there is no need to be open-minded or to search for truth once one has joined a particular group or after one has a religous experience. The ongoing search for truth is of ultimate importance in keeping a healthy spirituality.

Search for Truth—All religious founders and all great prophets have shown both by precept and by personal example the importance of the search for truth. They shared their experience of truth with others. In order for any belief system to have real effect, one has to internalize it or make it one's own.

Dermot Cox, a scripture scholar, explains the story of Job in the Old Testament from the point of view of the existential dilemma of human life. Job, unlike his fellow men, sets out to search for the meaning of his life and suffering. He entered into a dialogue with God but did not get any concrete and definite answers. He could not have said what is seen on many bumperstickers "I found it" and just held onto it. In his search for the ultimate answers, Job found his meaning in life and he lived authentically.

Others around him, the compliant religious people, used the illusory certainties of their religious tradition to calm their anxieties and shield themselves from facing the disturbing mystery of life. Job, on the other hand, set out to explore and experience the mystery as much as he, as a human being, could. Job experienced the importance of human consciousness as a source of meaning. He faced existential freedom and accepted the "absurdity" of life since we as human beings cannot grasp the entire scheme and meaning of life. In accepting this, he also went beyond the absurdity, and engaged himself in life. He chose "a way of life opposed to sin"; he chose light against darkness. In his search for God, Job went beyond the "essential" God or the "God of the philosophers" to the God known by experience.

> "Job, every man, knows that he will never attain the knowledge of God's ways with the world, but he also knows that by continually striving after the unknowable he will achieve human maturity."[2]

Rabbi Abraham Heschel makes a similar point: "[Thus] concealing the truth was necessary in order to make possible man's greatest adventure: to live in search. If truth had not been concealed, there would be no need to choose, to search."[3]

Buddha taught explicitly not to believe something just because a so-called wise man said it, or because it is written in an ancient holy book or because it is the popular belief. Buddha wanted individuals to use their own judgment with diligence, giving due consideration to authoritative sources of knowledge. One of the major thrusts of the teachings and examples of Jesus was to challenge the traditions of the time and open people's minds to an honest search for truth and love.

Paul Tillich pointed out two important ways people evade the search for truth in matters of significance: tradition and indifference.[4] Tradition can be a tragic perdition. It was more of a problem in the past. Indifference to truth is perhaps more of a problem in modern times. The alienation of people from nature and natural process in the industrialized countries, the rampant consumerism, and the lack of time for spiritual enrichment after the rat race for more material things, are major factors in the indifference of busy moderns.

Unhealthy adherence to tradition and indifference to truths that in any way challenge their rigid beliefs are important features of religious fanatics. Attachment to tradition is clearly irrational when it causes excessive fear, hate, or selfishness. Such irrational traditionalism also inevitably involves indifference to truth. Many of the conflicts between religion and science have been a result of religion's indifference to scientific truth. Even now, fundamentalists of various religions tend to deny scientific hypotheses or historical facts that go against their traditional beliefs. Some people, taking the biblical Genesis literally, believe that the world was created in six days.

As Mortimer J. Adler points out in *Six Great Ideas*, the search for truth in any branch of knowledge involves the addition of new truths, substitution of more accurate ideas or formulations in the place of less accurate ones, and discovery and correction of errors. It takes courage to go along with this process—something the fanatics lack. In the search for truth, we use reason and intuition. An important aspect of our reasoning is our questioning or doubting.

Reason and Doubt

Plato's definition of human beings as rational featherless bipeds may sound too cerebral and old fashioned. But who can question the uniqueness of human reason? No doubt Freudians and Existentialists have shown the importance of our irrational side. There is a method even in the madness of one's irrational side. In fact, the best blend is when the rational and the subconscious work in harmony.

Reason and doubt work together. In fact, researchers are systematic doubters and enquirers. What is healthy is not the paralyzing doubt of a perfectionist or the clever doubt of an attorney who doesn't care about the truth as much as winning his case. Genuine doubt is the handmaid of reason. These two have a proper place in spirituality—reason is encouraged and doubt accepted. Again, it takes courage and love to pursue reason, accept doubt in perspective, and act wholeheartedly in spite of the doubt.

Religious fanatics often consider human reason and doubt as evil tendencies. To doubt is to be damned; to reason is to go astray. "You just believe what we teach and live by it, or else God will get you," I was told by a well-educated and well-meaning woman who is a religious fanatic. The poet Tennyson has aptly declared: "There lives more faith in honest doubt, believe me, than in half your creeds."

Our unconscious has not only the depth of our instinctual but also the depth of our spiritual aspects as Viktor Frankl emphasized in *The Unconscious God*. Indeed it was a big mistake that Freud made to have seen only the instinctual aspect in the subconscious. Freudians can analyze away and reduce everything spiritual to be something instinctual—one of the high jinks of psychoanalysis. They are partially correct in so far as what may appear to be spiritual may not be genuinely spiritual; it may be coming from sexual and aggressive instincts. For example, I have come across innumerable instances of religious fanatics claiming genuine compassion and love for others only to mask their need to control and use others for their own selfish needs.

To give one example, an older married minister had an affair with a young married woman. He continued to pretend that he was trying to help her because of genuine love. Whenever she expressed her doubt and guilt over the affair, he reassured her saying that he had prayed about it and it was okay. He also convinced her that he was leading her closer to Divine Love. This woman was faced with fear of death on one occasion, accidentally, and then all her fears and guilt surfaced. She made a serious suicide attempt but survived. During therapy it was clear that she had abandoned her own reasoning and love under the strong influence of a minister who was pursuing his instinctual drives in the name of spirituality.

So, we have to use our common sense and our reasoning power to decide whether what is coming from our subconscious is genuinely spiritual or the wolf of our instincts dressed up as the sheep of spirituality. That is possible only if we keep an open mind—not if we are closed minded.

Open and Closed Mind

Milton Rokeach's book *The Open and Closed Mind* is the best source on the subject that I have discovered. He has shown the important elements of the closed and open belief systems. His findings are very useful for a clear understanding of the healthy and unhealthy dynamics of religion.

Any belief system consists of several subsystems and a disbelief system. The open-minded system shows communication and consistency between subsystems and belief/disbelief systems. On the other hand, the closed mind shows compartmentalization and inconsistency of subsystems or belief/disbelief systems. For example, a closed-minded person may claim to be a staunch supporter of democracy and a strong opponent of totalitarianism. However, he/she may support oligarchies or military dictatorships because of personal economic gain and continue to deny the inconsistency with various rationalizations. Rokeach also observes that the open-belief system showed much less intensity in the rejection of the disbelief system compared to the intensity with which closed minds rejected disbelief systems.

The open mind has an outlook of friendliness toward the world, whereas the closed mind has an outlook of threat. People with the more open belief system do not rely excessively on authority, whereas people with a relatively closed belief system rely heavily on authority and judge other people on the basis of the latter's reliance (or otherwise) on the same authority. While the open-minded person has high ability to evaluate information on its own merits, closed-minded persons show poor ability to do so. The closed-minded individuals depend on authority to make the decisions for them. An extension of this process is even more interesting: people with closed minds tend to swallow whatever the accepted authority says, even if it is contradictory to the other belief systems they hold. Open-minded people cannot be "taken for a ride" by authority because they use their own judgment and look for consistency.

There are two very powerful motivations that underlie the belief/disbelief systems. One of these is the need to know and understand; the other factor is the need to protect oneself from any threatening aspect of reality. The stronger the need to know and understand—and the weaker the need to ward off threats—the more open is the resulting system. The stronger the need to protect from the threat of reality, the more closed the system becomes. In short, an individual is as open to knowledge as possible and as closed to knowledge as necessary (as necessary, based on the person's fear). The person with a closed mind tries to overcome insecurity and self-hate by over-identifying with the authority figure. This is different from accepting a great person as one's ideal or one's model to follow.

Interestingly, closed-minded people have less memory of any information that may challenge or refute their belief system. This is because of their unwillingness to play along and not reject a challenging idea outright. The capacity for synthesis is strong in open-minded individuals and is very weak in the closed-minded ones. Also, closed-minded persons have much greater difficulty in forming new conceptual and perceptual systems. Those who scored high on dogmatism scales were also the ones who scored high on anxiety scales in Rokeach's studies. Evaluation of a dozen ecumenical councils of the Catholic Church were interesting: the more threatening the situation was before convening the council, the more absolute and prohibitive were the canons enacted by the council.

Rokeach's above findings are applicable to individuals with unhealthy religiosity. Religious fanatics have extremely closed belief systems. But healthy spiritiuality and open-mindedness go hand in hand.

Prejudice—William James observed that piety can be a mask covering up the tribal instincts of rejecting outsiders. Because of space limitations I do not want to get into various aspects of prejudice. For anyone interested in reading more on the subject I recommend Gordon Allport's book *The Nature of Prejudice*. A few of Allport's ideas will be considered here.

There are different degrees of negative action that are manifested as a result of prejudice. It may be expresed in talking badly about the objects of prejudice, usually in conversation with like-minded people. A further level of prejudice is manifested in avoidance of the disliked group. One degree worse is discrimination. And when prejudice is even more intense, it leads to physical attack and ultimately to extermination.

Allport quite rightly concludes that prejudice has multiple causes. An historical cause of prejudice is rationalization of the exploitation of one group by another; for example, the colonialist's argument that the colonial subjects were inferior and in need of protection. Sociological factors of prejudice include differences of the traditions of various groups, the type of interaction and communication between groups, and relative rootlessness associated with urbanization. Situational causes of prejudice include unemployment and other fnancial pressures. Psychodynamic factors involve frustration of the person's needs and insecure or authoritarian personality. Stereotyping and earned negative reputation are other factors. Allport noted the paradoxical position of religion: it can cause prejudice or it can help to eliminate prejudice.

As to why religion causes prejudice, Allport says: "The chief reason why religion becomes the focus of prejudice is that it usually stands for more than faith—it is the pivot of the cultural tradition of the group."[5]

Religious leaders of a community often rationalize, uphold, and sanctify the secular practices of their followers. Not infrequently the more vehemently the leader does it, the more respect and power he gets from the group. Leaders who crave power and position can easily manipulate these dynamics. Allport and others have shown that people whose religion is interiorized (or those who make use of religion for personal growth) are, in fact, far less prejudiced than the average individual. On the other hand, those who find a safe and secure haven in the religious institution and identify with its powerful in group are highly prejudiced.

Prejudice is pre-judging. While the tendency to pre-judge is not healthy, we have to make judgments to make decisions and take steps. And we have to judge our own actions. That brings us to the issue of conscience or moral reasoning.

Conscience—According to psychoanalysis, our superego is formed in childhood by the internalization of the prohibitions and commands of our parents or parent substitutes. Then, it modifies as we emulate other people outside the family. The proper function of the conscience is to warn the ego to do what is right and avoid the pain of guilt. Hamlet said that conscience makes cowards of us all. Healthy conscience makes us only prudent, not cowardly. However, too rigid and strict a conscience can make us not only cowards but very miserable with guilt, resulting in depression.

Conscience is a self-monitoring process. Bernard Lonergan describes four successive levels of conscience which are inter-related. The first is the empirical level at which we perceive and speak. The second, the intellectual level, is where we make inquiries and develop understanding and express what we understand. On the third, the rational level, we reason and reflect on the evidence and then make a judgment. Finally, on the fourth, the responsible level, we decide on the possible course of action and carry it out.[6] These levels explain the process of our self-monitoring and not the level of maturity of the conscience. As far as the stages of maturation of our conscience are concerned, the six stages of moral reasoning by Lawrence Kohlberg are very pertinent.

Kohlberg divided the six stages into three levels. At level one, the *preconventional level*, the child (or the grown-up who is fixated at this level) follows cultural notions of good and bad because of the practical consequences of reward/punishment or exchange of favors. Level one has two stages:

—Stage one manifests the punishment and obedience orientation in which the goodness or badness of actions is based on reward or punishment that results from the action. For example, an action is deemed bad solely because the person got punished for it.

—Stage two of the preconventional level shows instrumental purpose and equal exchange orientation. Here what is right is what action meets one's needs. If a favor is done, it is with the purpose of the other person's meeting one's own need in return. Therefore it is the value system of the market place.

On the next level, the *conventional level*, the person follows the expectations of his group (family, nation, and so on). What is good is what is approved by the group and what is bad is what the group disapproves, regardless other aspects of the matter. There is strong loyalty to the group. There are, again, two stages in this level.

—The first stage (stage three of moral reasoning) is of good boy/nice girl orientation where one behaves according to group norms and gains the acceptance of others as being nice.

—The next stage, stage four, is the stage of social system and conscience maintenance, in which obeying rules is seen as right behavior and maintaining social order is of prime importance, not for its higher purposes but for its own sake.

On the next level, the *post-conventional level*, the person's moral evaluation goes beyond the authority of one's groups. There are two stages here, too.

—The fifth stage of moral reasoning is the social-contract legalistic orientation. It has a utilitarian flavor. A person at this stage is willing to change his/her value system based on rational considerations of the utility of the value system for the society. This is in contrast to rigid adherence to the given value system as in stage four. What is right or wrong is decided by critical evaluation and free agreements, and contracts become binding, with a sense of obligation.

—The sixth stage is that of universal ethical principle. At this stage what is right or wrong is decided on the basis of ethical principles that utilize critical reasoning, universality, and consistency. The Golden Rule is a good example of such ethical principle.[7]

The moral reasoning of people with unhealthy religiosity is of the first four stages, especially the first two. Not surprisingly, the moral reasoning of healthy spirituality is of stages five and six. For example, religious fanatics often expect divine blessing just from performing a ritual even though they (fanatics) may be violating the spirit of love and goodness. For a caste-ridden Hindu, following the unjust practices of his caste is right because his community approves it. Similarly, the racist Christian. When Jesus said that the Sabbath was made for man and not man made for the Sabbath, He was showing post-conventional moral reasoning. However, someone who is fixated at the conventional level of conscience would disagree with such statements; this person would probably predict gloom and doom if people do not strictly adhere to the laws and traditions. Someone on a preconventional level would be frightened of divine retribution for not observing the Sabbath.

Consciences that are based on reward/punishment or marketing values can be easily corrupted. Hence the inconsistency in their actions and their guilt. Fundamentalist Christians fear that, if the Bible is not held as inerrant, then everyone would interpret it as he or she pleases, resulting in terrible confusion. This is an example of the extreme fear of people functioning on lower levels of conscience who do not understand the higher level of conscience. Even the fact that millions of Christians who do not believe in the total inerrancy of the Bible live good Christian lives is not impressive to these people.

The psychological dynamics behind the preconventional level of moral reasoning, I believe, are fear and selfish interests. The dynamics of the conventional level of conscience is largely that of group identification. At the post-conventional level, the dynamic forces are love, wisdom, and courage/ prudence.

Intuition—The word intuition originated from the Latin word *intueri* which means "to look at or contemplate." It is the knowing that bypasses the usual rational process—an integral part of the mystical experience. Some people seem to think anybody who is eccentric but not psychotic and is deeply involved with religion is a mystic. These are wrong impressions. Intuitive knowledge is not deductive but inductive. It is not opposed to sense perception and logic but goes beyond it.

Intuition has been given tremendous importance in Eastern religions. Much of the religious training in various schools of mysticism helps to develop this capacity. Some of the Western misunderstanding of the East is attributable to the Eastern emphasis on intuition which is seen as antirational, life-denying, withdrawal into oneself, and the like. Indeed, such negative extremes do happen but that is not true intuition.

In the Western mystical tradition, too, intuition has been held high. From early Church Fathers through medieval mystics to Thomas Merton in this century, the Christian mystics have carried on the tradition of contemplation and the development of intuitive knowledge.Similarly,Jewish and Islamic mystics, notably followers of Hasidism and Sufism respectively, have been great proponents of intuitive knowledge.

Many great Western thinkers have been staunch advocates of intuition. Socrates believed that our soul has been born several times and much of our knowledge is recollection. Such recollection is intuitive. Plato's idea of penetrating the shadowy world of appearances and seeing the true light of life is akin to mystical wisdom. Aristotle considered contemplation the highest of all activities, in sharp contrast to a modern impression of contemplation as extreme passivity. Spinoza, Bergson, and Pascal are among other great thinkers who recognized the role of intuition.

Modern physics has moved away from the mechanistic and fragmented views of Newtonian physics. Writers such as Capra, Lesham, Talbot, and Zukav have drawn parallels between mystical insights of religions and the scientific insights of modern physics. Fritjof Capra, a physicist, notes that the mystic who starts from the inner world and the physicist who starts from the outer world reach similar conclusions. He observes: "the harmony between their views confirms the ancient Indian wisdom that Brahman, the ultimate reality without, is identical to Atman, the reality within."[8] Reflective of the new outlook is the famous statement of Sir James Jeans as to the universe looking like a great thought rather than a great machine.

Carl Jung gave much importance to intuition both in his practice and in his writings. He saw the function of intuition as perceiving the interconnectedness and relationships of events and entities. Jung's idea of synchronicity is particlarly interesting. Synchronicity means a connection between the meaning of two events. It is not just coincidence; it is coincidence with meaning. Therefore, it is the subjective experience of a person. The meaning of the events links together in the human psyche.

Along with the interconnectedness is another important aspect of intuition—self-reflection. This is a power of the human mind as important, or more so, than our capacity for reasoning. While reasoning is a conscious process, self-reflection is as much a subconscious process also. Saying that the subconscious walks a yard in front of us indicates the usefulness of the intuitive process.

One has to bear in mind the potential for harm in pursuing intuition at the expense of reason. By throwing reason and common sense out the window, the pursuers of imaginary intuition become increasingly less in touch with reality. Religious cults provide plenty of examples of such destructive deviation from the human potential of intuition. That brings us to the psychology of self-deception.

Psychology of Self-Deception

In his book on the psychology of self-deception, *Vital Lies, Simple Truths*, Daniel Goleman gives a good overview of the up-to-date understanding on the subject, particularly on the basis of studies by cognitive psychologists in recent times. He draws three important conclusions:

A. By reducing awareness, the mind can protect itself from anxiety.

B. This process leads to blind spots. These are areas of darkness and self-deception.

C. These areas of darkness occur at every major level of behavior on individual and social levels.

Psychological defenses are varieties of self-deception. What is the purpose of dimming awareness and thereby reducing pain? It is a survival mechanism. If we are paralyzed by fear, we would not be able to face challenges and threats. Being alert to dangers is essential for our survival. At the extreme end of the continuum of arousal is anxiety.

Information is transformed, not just transmitted, as it passes through the mind. The information that we perceive is scanned and filtered before it reaches our awareness. Therefore what reaches our awareness is not the whole truth; in fact, it can be so modified that it may have little resemblance to the truth. Our long-term memory, based on our experiences in life up to the moment, plays the decisive role in scanning and filtering the information. Wishful thinking and egocentricity have a very strong influence in the scanning and filtering processes. Long-term memories themselves are modified in ways to suit these two factors. Information that is threatening to self-esteem is modified in different ways. People who have depressive tendencies perceive and take seriously the information that lowers their self-esteem whereas more cheerful people reduce both the perception and the significance of such information.

Various of Goleman's ideas set forth above, are also expressed by literary figures. As Dostoevsky's famous hero—the Underground Man in *Notes from Underground*—observed, there are some secrets that a man would tell only his friends, other matters he would tell only himself, and still other things he would not even tell himself. This game of secrets goes on within the individual and between individuals and in various groups such as families, communities, and nations. Henrik Ibsen wrote about the family pretenses. Being quite aware of the significance of the game, Ibsen stated that if we rob an ordinary person of his "vital lie" we would be depriving him of his happiness.

Interconnectedness of Knowledge with Love and Courage

There is a very definite and strong connection between love and truth. Paul Tillich noted this connection and advised us strongly to distrust any claim of truth where we can observe the lack of love. Love is no secret mystery but something that has clearly observable manifestations. I say this because people with unhealthy religiosity often claim to love but really show indifference or hate. They can only fool themselves and others with similar problems; any insightful person can make out their compartmentalization or hypocrisy. Courage and prudence are very much a part of open-mindedness. Open-mindedness reinforces courage and prudence by the true knowledge the person gains. Also, in its turn, the additional knowledge reinforces courage and prudence. As fear lessens, so love increases.

Wisdom—In these days of increasing cleverness, not much is heard of wisdom—we may be becoming too clever to be wise. However, the concept of wisdom is a jewel in the crown of religion. *Wisdom involves knowledge, openmindedness, post-conventional level of conscience, and a balance between reason and intuition.* With these comes also a universal identity.

Paul Tillich describes wisdom beautifully: "It is insight into the meaning of one's life, into its conflicts and dangers, into its creative and destructive powers, and into the ground out of which it comes and to which it must return."[9]

Tillich emphasized the importance of the statement in the Bible: "The fear of the Lord is the beginning of wisdom, and the knowledge of the holy is understanding." A sense of awe at the mystery of life is an integral part of wisdom. It is interesting to note how Christian fanatics emphasize the first part of this statement without even conceding that fear is only the *beginning* of wisdom.

In June 1985, *Psychology Today* published an interesting survey (by Laurer & Laurer) of couples who have been married for fifteen years or more. Among the top four reasons given by them for their lasting relationship was a sense of sacredness about marriage. So, it is obvious that the sense of sacredness is quite valuable. Sadly, we may be losing it fast with the kind of consumerism that is devouring us. In marriage itself, and in other relationships, the sense of sacredness is fast eroding. A junior resident, a woman doctor, said she did not see any sacredness in her relationship with her live-in boyfriend. She prided herself over her scientific bent that kept her from being stupid like the people who consider intimate relations sacred. It is understandable that many people are revolting against the superstitious extremes to which the sense of sacredness was side-tracked in the past.

Knowledge without wisdom degenerates into selfish manipulation, alienation, and destruction of self and others. This is seen in all types of exploitation where the victimizer knows how to take advantage of the victim. The same happens with unhealthy religiosity. Healthy spirituality channels knowledge toward wisdom. Attainment of wisdom—"vidya" in Hinduism, and "prajna" in Buddhism—is one of the highest goals of spiritual life of all peoples. Observed Jungian analyst and Episcopalian priest, John A. Sanford: "All true morality springs from the clarity of consciousness. All else is done in darkness and leads to distortions, not to love."[10] An integral part of our self-awareness is our sense of identity. The way religion fosters identity conflicts or helps to form holistic, well-integrated identity will be dealt with in the next chapter.

10. IDENTITY

*"He who begins by loving Christianity better than
Truth, will proceed by loving his own sect or church
better than Christianity and end in loving himself
better than them all."* — Coleridge

*"I am not an Athenian or a Greek but a citizen of
the world."* — Socrates

In an interesting instance, a young man suffered from a brief psychosis related to an identity problem. Tom, in his early twenties, sought help because he felt people were staring at him and spreading rumor that he was a homosexual. He also heard some voices accusing him of being a 'faggot'. All these symptoms started after an argument with his girl friend who used her sharp tongue and accused him of being a 'sissy' and a 'fruitcake'. She obviously knew that would hurt him most and he apparently had not heeded the Bard's warning against unbelieving priests, dull teachers, and sharp tongued women.

He was a macho male who believed in being the real man. He played football, enjoyed hunting and collecting knives and guns, got intoxicated on Friday and Saturday nights, and did womanize occasionally although he and his girl friend were engaged. His girl friend was irate about his flirting with other girls but she accused him of being a 'sissy' and a 'fruitcake' instead. Tom had grown up in an insecure family situation because of an almost absent father. He did not have a strong religious identity. The lukewarm religious identity he had was that of 'muscular Christianity' wth a belief in the power of Christian nations. Treatment with antipsychotic medications cured his psychotic symptoms in about two weeks. And psychotherapy helped him to gain insight into his shaky masculine identity which was being covered up with machismo. As he became really strong, he gave up his mask.

We hear a lot about identity: national identity, ethnic identity, changing identity, gender identity, identity crisis, and so on. It might even appear to be a modern discovery. The psychological and sociological theories and studies are something new. However, the issues of identity have been religious concerns for millenniums before these new developments. Identity is a central theme in Hinduism, one of the oldest religions of the world.

S. Radhakrishnan said: "Brahman, the first principle of the universe, is known through atman, the inner self of man."[1] "Narayana is the God in man who lives in constant association with nara, the human being. He is the immortal dwelling in the mortals."[2] And in Hinduism the ultimate goal is to attain true knowledge of the divine in us which is part of the Brahman. That is our true identity but our ignorance (*avidya*) causes false identity and unhappy consequences from it.

It is not only man that shows evidence of a sense of identity. Many species of animal show a pecking order of status in the group. Similarly, territorial rights are important for many species and they are ready to fight to defend these rights.

Zoologists and ethologists note several advantages in having a pecking order. It helps to minimize intraspecies aggression; it also helps the species to survive adverse conditions such as shortage of food when the strong ones feed and the weak ones starve. As the dominant males in many species have more access to mate, the survival of the fittest is favored.

Identity and Identity Problems in Man

According to one of Plato's myths, before birth people choose the lives they will live. But then they drink the waters of Lethe which is the river of forgetfulness. After birth they identify themselves with their roles in life and live unaware of the deeper dimensions of their selfhood. Plato taught that people can be awakened from this state and can attain a state of nonforgetfulness (alethia) through good insight.

The word 'identity' is derived from the Latin word 'idem' meaning 'self-sameness'. Psychoanalyst Erik Erikson has contributed immensely to our understanding of identity and related issues. Identity is almost as central to Erikson as sexuality was to Freud. Erikson says: "A sense of identity means a sense of being at one with oneself as one grows and develops; and it means, at the same time, a sense of affinity with a community's sense of being at one with its future as well as its history or mythology."[3]

Human development proceeds by stages and each stage has its particular task. Erikson formulates eight stages of life, in which the adolescent stage faces the individual with "identity versus identity confusion." During adolescence, individuals sense more clearly their uniqueness as people and at the same time experience more intensely their relatedness to a larger whole. They become aware of inherent characteristics, physical and mental features and boundaries. They experience a variety of issues relating to friendship, sexual orientation, career, group loyalties, value systems, and religious identification. The maturing ego of the adolescent has the capacity to integrate these into a healthy whole. When such integration is in trouble, identity confusion results. Identity confusion can leave the adolescent feeling anxious, empty, confused, isolated, and indecisive. Successful completion of the previous stages of life as well as stable and supportive family and social environment help the adolescent greatly to develop healthy identity.

Negative identity is one of the problems that results when the process of identity goes wrong. It refers to the sense of having bad or unworthy characteristics. The old saying that a child or a dog will live up to or down to its reputation is very true. Not only that, one may project the negative identity onto others, leading to prejudices. A young man with personality disorder whom I treated was extremely prejudiced against blacks and homosexuals. He himself had all the characteristics of unreliability and high emotionality which he was accusing the blacks of. He was insecure in his masculine identity and masked it by playing macho, even abusing his wife.

Erikson's concepts of 'wholeness', 'totalism', and 'pseudospeciation' are very useful for our purpose. In his own words: "As a Gestalt, then, wholeness emphasizes a sound, organic, progressive mutuality between diversified functions and parts within an entirety, the boundaries of which are open and fluid. Totality, on the contrary, evokes a Gestalt in which absolute boundary is emphasized. Given a certain arbitrary delineation, nothing that belongs inside must be left outside, nothing that must be outside can be tolerated inside."[4]

High levels of integration allow greater diversity and more tolerance of tensions; low levels of integration maintain a sense of security by totalities and conformities. Erikson's concept of 'pseudospeciation' refers to the human tendency to behave as different species. "The *pseudo* means that, far from perceiving or accepting a human identity based on a common species-hood, different tribes and nations, creeds and classes (and perchance political parties) consider themselves to be the one chosen species and will, especially in times of crisis, sacrifice to this claim much of the knowledge, the logic, and the ethics that are theirs."[5]

Intraspecies aggression is minimal in the animal kingdom. But it is highly prevalent in human beings, to a great extent because of pseudospeciation. Conflict between different groups is a good example. All wars fall into this category. If other species knew about the way mankind fights, they might laugh or cry themselves to death!

Identity and religion

In his scholarly work *Identity and the Sacred*, Hans Mol defines religion as the 'sacralization' of identity. By sacralization he means "the process of becoming or making sacred."[6] He shows how religion sacralizes individual and social identity and thereby provides an extremely useful function. Mol attempts to integrate the approaches of various schools on religion—anthropology, history, psychology, and sociology.

Mol points out that in animals and man order gives security and has survival value. At the same time, too much order means less adaptation and another kind of danger. Individual identity is the stable niche that a person occupies in a rather chaotic environment. Social identity is a stable combination of common beliefs and patterns of behavior. Both the individual and the group defend their identity from various threats. Prejudice is an important method of fostering group identity by protecting it from external threats. Taboos do the same.

There is interdependence as well as conflicts between personal and group identities. Both types of identity are strengthened by art, play, and religion. Mol gives conversion as an example of identity formation on a personal level. New converts have new identities and often they try to reinforce the new identity and denounce the old one. Witnessing reinforces the new identity of the convert as well as strengthens the affiliation of the group. This dynamic is effectively utilized by self-help groups such as "Alcoholics Anonymous." Change of identity involves change of one's outlook on oneself, one's role in activities, and one's reference group. The vigorous enthusiasm of the new convert in spreading his new faith is well known.

An example of religion influencing social identity is provided by charismatic religious leaders. Acting as catalysts for social change, they forge a new social identity. The new identity and the changes that come with it may be for better or worse, as our examples of Gandhi and of Jim Jones will show.

Morality and identity are closely linked—the former being what is expected of a person or society and the latter being what the individual or group essentially is.

There are various foci of identity such as family, class, caste, sex, and nation. Religion tends to make these sacred. Family is particularly important as a focus of identity. Centuries before all the theories about families and therapies for their problems, religion worked to enhance family ties and obligations. In Hinduism it is after the stage of family obligations that the stages of sagehood are entered. The importance given to family by religions continues even in our times of crisis in family relationships. The statement that the family that prays together stays together is relevant in many ways.

Several studies have shown that rituals, particularly rites of passage, are followed even by people who have very little connection to organized religion otherwise. In some European countries and in Australia where a good percentage of people are not regular churchgoers, baptism, weddings, and funerals are still important functions in church for almost all. There is a saying that even the irreligious go to church three times—once walking and twice being carried.

Identity in Religious Fanatics

Fanatics show 'totality' and 'pseudospeciation'. The true believers are inside the boundary and all the rest are outside. There is a tendency to look down on, dislike, or even hate the outsiders. There may even be a sort of indifference with a shade of hostility. However, the dislike and hatred of the black sheep within the group itself is at least equally intense.

A sense of the group's superiority is fostered. In trying to rationalize pride, the individual or group focuses on some real or imagined features which are considered superior to others. It may be one's geographical area, mother tongue, color of skin, and/or religious beliefs and practices. If there is some real achievement in some aspect of life, it is often taken out of perspective in order to keep up an unhealthy pride. Sometimes the focus of pride is based on history. In order to keep the sense of superiority, people readily overlook or distort reality. It is interesting to listen to some religious leaders denounce their own country for various evils and warn about dire consequences, and in the next breath glorify the same country as God's favorite nation.

Negative identity and conflict over several aspects of identity are obvious in unhealthy religiosity. Rather than modify and integrate the shadow side, the undesirable aspects are often projected onto others. Then, of course, the next step is to convert or destroy the other. Thus men or women with sexual identity conflicts may become intensely hateful toward homosexuals. In trying to disprove the presence of some conflict in sexual identity, men may develop a macho personality and women a hysterical personality—caricatures of the masculine and feminine roles respectively. Psychological studies have shown that 'androgynous' individuals—those who combine masculine and feminine qualities—are healthier than others in their identity.

Negative identity projected onto others becomes prejudice. Pride and prejudice are caused by—and maintained with—ignorance. The Orwellian formula "ignorance is strength" is implicit under the facade that everything worth knowing is within the group's ideology. On many occasions, I have tried to give some information very matter-of-factly, without any tinge of criticism, to religious fanatics; and on all such occassions it was received with varying degrees of hostility.

Religious extremists tend to give excessive importance to narrow foci of identity such as gender, caste, race, and nationality, at the expense of a universal identity. In all the notable hotbeds of religious conflict, regionalism is an important factor. For example, the struggle in Northern Ireland, the militancy of Sikh extremists in India, and the Iran-Iraq war are motivated by religious identity combined with regional identity. When religion sanctifies a focus of identity, the latter gains great status. The Hindu organization R. S. S. (Rashtriya Swayamsewak Sangh) in India has a revealing formula—"Hindu, Hindi, Hindustani." It clearly rhymes well but the reasoning behind it is an unfortunate narrowing, rigidification, and exclusiveness of Indian identity with Hindu religion and Hindi language. Sanctification of ethnicity causes pseudospeciation. For example, a Christian minister revived the KKK in the U.S. in 1915 with the slogan, "Protestant Christianity and White Supremacy."

Sexual identity is an important part of a person's overall identity. Male chauvinism has been an unfortunate part of religious tradition in the East and the West. However, in the depths of these religions, one can discern holistic identity. In *Identity* Ruth Tiffany Barnhouse points out that in the Old Testament God's reaching out to his people is often described in feminine terms, e.g. using the feminine word *yad* (hand). Similarly the Sanskrit word *Sakti*, representing the active aspect of deity, is also a feminine noun. Meister Eckhart referred to creation as God giving birth.

Psychiatry has not had the *guts* to include macho personality within the classification of personality disorders. Nonetheless, it is one of the worst personality problems. The macho male tends to be too aggressive; too superficial; and too unwilling to negotiate, to understand, to grow and mature emotionally and spiritually. The admiration for many such characters, even in modern societies, is an indication of the vast room for growth that still remains. The Belgian Association of Safe Driving has come up with some clever advertisements to influence the "macho" male. In one of those advertisements, a beautiful blonde says: "Fast driving is as stupid as fast love-making." And in another ad, the poster girl goes even further: "You can't seduce me if you drive fast."

Unhealthy religiosity tends to sanctify narrow notions of masculinity and femininity. We dealt with the issue of women wearing pants earlier in the book. There are some aggressive Christian fundamentalists who argue that Jesus was not a 'wimp'. They point out the few examples when Jesus used force to support their case. One prominent TV evangelist identifies with the image of "strongman" Jesus who took out the whip and overturned the tables in the Temple, angry with the people who were trading in the place of worship. For this evangelist, the "wimpy" looking Jesus "patting the back of puny little billy goats" is not the real Jesus. In fact they imply that Jesus was a macho man. That is totally false. Jesus was not at all a macho man. Christian mystics like Julian of Norwich and Anselm of Canterbury referred to Jesus as our Mother. In fact, Jesus showed a universal identity of personhood above the macho and wimp categories. The issue of homosexuality and religion is particularly revealing. Most of the male homosexuals I have treated have come from fundamentalistic religious families with heavy emphasis on macho masculinity. The fathers of these patients were rough and tough, often neglecting or mistreating their women. The sensitive sons could not identify with the fathers. The father of one patient—a fundamentalist and a police officer—threatened to kill the son if the latter did not change sexual orientation. (The son did not change but kept away from the father.) Thus, ironically, fundamentalists appear to contribute to the causation of homosexuality which they vehemently condemn.

A sharply delineated and vehemently defended identity has temporary usefulness. As those who are weak may need some crutches, those with identity problems may temporarily benefit from the fanatical kind of identity. It is not surprising that young people struggling with identity conflicts are prime candidates to join fanatical groups. As studies of religious cults show, the need for believing and belonging may be met by fanatical groups. Studies of presidential assassins reveal that they have significant identity confusion and often use aliases. They often ally with extremist groups of right-wing or left-wing political persuasion. Such alliance must be meeting the need for identity. The danger is fixation at that level and further worsening of the condition.

Fear of losing identity is at the root of intolerance and fear of dialogue. Some well-known fundamentalist writers are quoted as declaring, "The danger of tolerance is that ultimately the movement will lose its identity and will begin to drift toward the position of the people with whom it carries on a dialogue."[7] Healthy spirituality provides courage to face such fears.

Identity in Mature Spirituality

We noted earlier that the issue of our true identity is central to Hinduism. Similarly Buddhists talk about our original face and Taoists speak of our original nature. As Albert Nolan points out, "Jesus' frequent and emphatic use of the term 'Son of Man' was his way of referring to and identifying himself with man as man."[8]

Aldous Huxley's views about the deeper aspect of religions illustrate the close connections between universal identity and mature spirituality. According to Huxley, underneath all the apparent differences in outlook and expression of the world religions there is a "Highest Common Factor" which is the "Perennial

Philosophy." He finds four fundamental doctrines at the core of the perennial philosophy:

"First: The phenomenal world of matter and of individualized consciousness—the world of things and animals and men and even gods—is the manifestation of a Divine Ground within which all partial realities have their being, and apart from which they would be nonexistent.

Second: Human beings are capable not merely of knowing *about* the Divine Ground by inference; they can also realize its existence by a direct intuition, superior to discursive reasoning. This immediate knowledge unites the knower with that which is known.

Third: Man possesses a double nature, a phenomenal ego and an eternal Self, which is the inner man, the spirit, the spark of divinity within the soul. It is possible for a man, if he so desires, to identify himself with the spirit and therefore with the Divine Ground, which is of the same or like nature with the spirit.

Fourth: Man's life on earth has only one end and purpose: to identify himself with his eternal Self and so to come to unitive knowledge of the Divine Ground."[9]

Mature spirituality works toward larger, more inclusive identities. Even as the various foci of identity such as sex, nationality, and ethnic group are given their own importance, much more importance is given to the deeper self. Jesus told his followers to give to Caesar what is his and to give to God what is His. Religious fanatics tend to give God money through religious organizations and to give the State or some such foci of identity their everyday allegiance.

As our deepest being, our own eternal Self, becomes the primary focus of our identity, other aspects of identity fall into place. This does not mean there are no conflicts or weaknesses in these other foci of identity. There may be conflicts, but the conflicts are dealt with more easily. In my clinical experience this has been very true. For example, conflicts relating to sexual identity were much more easily resolved in people with a healthy centering of identity on their deeper self compared to the same conflicts in people whose identities are centered on some other foci such as profession, gender, and nationality.

The reason that spiritually mature people are only minimally prejudiced is because they do not need such defenses. Negative identity may not be significantly present; or, if it is there, it is integrated into the larger whole rather than projected onto others.

All the great religions of the world on their healthy side foster a universal identity. However, their followers often overlook this and identify wrongly with region, class, race, and the like. For example, Prophet Mohammed became an eminent leader at a time when the divisions and strifes of various groups had made human life miserable in his part of the world. The plight of women was especially bad. With Prophet Mohammed's leadership, a new unity and broad identity arose. As history shows and as we witness today, that identity and unity did not last too long; the split in Islam created new foci of identity and new cause for conflict and destruction. Jesus repeatedly emphasized his solidarity with the whole of mankind. Gandhi frequently emphasized the fact that whether Christian, Hindu, Jew, Moslem, or otherwise, we are all children of the one and the same God. As great a national leader as Gandhi was, he clearly saw that to do good to one's own nation—to be a loyal citizen of one's country—does not mean one's focus of identity has to be primarily one's nationality. Nor was Socrates a traitor in claiming to be a world citizen rather than an Athenian or a Greek. It is interesting how Jesus pointed to the Seal of Caesar on the coin and advised giving to Caesar what was his. Healthy loyalty to one's community and nation does not contradict a genuine universal identity.

When the Buddha heard that his kinsmen Sakyas and another group of people (the Kolis) were on the verge of battle over water rights, he did not bless his side. He explored the real reason for the conflict and exposed the folly of fighting over water which they admitted was less important than human lives. Similarly in the 16th Century when Spain was colonizing Latin America and destroying the native Indians, christian apologists argued that Indians were "natural slaves" to justify the action. But genuinely Christian missionaries like Bertalome' de Las Casas stood firmly against such hypocrisy and pointed out the evil nature of Spanish exploitation and destruction of the Indians.

Identities of Buddha and Las Casas were obviously beyond their group loyalties. Many religious leaders lack such holistic identities and tend to support and sanctify their community's unreasonable positions. And many moderate individuals support or sympathise with extremists of their religion because of the common religious identity. This only makes matters worse by strengthening the extremists.

Obligations and commitments to the various groups have definite importance in our lives. For, like it or not, we are social animals. However, the ultimate loyalty to the Creator and identification with our deepest self and its connectedness to the ground of Being is above and beyond all the other loyalties and identifications. This is the attitude of the spiritually mature.

Rollo May makes a very pertinent statement about moralism in his book *Discovery of Being*: "Indeed, compulsive and rigid moralism arises in given persons precisely as the result of a lack of sense of being."[10] He further explains such moralism as a mechanism of compensation—the lack of inner authority is compensated by overemphasis on external authority. A sense of being gives the person a basis for self-esteem not dependent on other people's opinions. Ego is only a part of our personality, the conscious part that tries to meet the demands from four masters—the Id, the superego, the external world, and a super consciousness (or intuition). The sense of being involves our whole experience—both conscious and unconscious.

One of the most important factors that prevents us from developing the sense of being is the 'having' orientation in life. Erich Fromm devoted a whole book to this issue. In *To Have or to Be*, Fromm contrasts the 'being mode' of life and the 'having mode' of life. Happiness of a person with a 'having mode' of life depends on superiority and power over others including the capacity to exploit, dominate, and destroy. In sharp contrast, happiness in the 'being mode' lies in caring, sharing and loving. Thus asceticism is not what Fromm has in mind when he opposes the 'having mode'; in fact, he explains that asceticism may be a cover-up for a 'having mode' deep down. A Buddhist once told me: "One of the worst attachments can be the attachment to the appearance of detachment."

Fromm approves of 'existential having'—having things that we need for our existence. What he opposes is what he calls 'characteriological having', a socially conditioned, passionate drive for things. Unfortunately, these points are not sufficiently elaborated. Meister Eckhart, the great Christian mystic, was strongly opposed to "merchant mentality," as are great teachers of other faiths.

In my view, 'having' that is consistent with love, courage/prudence, and wisdom is healthy. On the other hand 'having' that is from egoism, narcissism, hate, excessive fear, or lack of prudence is unhealthy. For example, having an efficiently running car that helps me to do my work instead of wasting time, energy, and resources for repairs is good. But, if I buy the sales pitch of the advertisers and become the *'proud owner'* of a prestigious model car, and my caring for this car takes me away from my work and family, then it is certainly unhealthy. It is even worse if my own identity is focused on being the owner of this car. Similarly identifying oneself with status symbols can work against a healthy holistic identity.

We tend to love and cherish that with which we identify. The narrowing of our love, as Coleridge pointed out [in the quotation at the beginning of the chapter], happens easily with the narrowing of identity. The broader the identity, the broader the love. Thus mature spirituality fosters 'wholeness' while unhealthy religiosity fosters 'totalism' and 'pseudospeciation', to use Erikson's terms.

Much of human conflict and consequent suffering—much of the inhumanity of human beings to one another—has been due to identity conflicts. More than at any other time in history, we have the opportunity to understand and correct it. The big question is whether we will do that or whether we will continue in our old ways. Religion can sprinkle holy water on destructive tendencies in identity, or it can lead us onto the constructive path of holistic identity. *Ultimately, the healthy identity involves the harmonious union of uniqueness and unity.* Healthy spirituality fosters the process; unhealthy religiosity hinders it.

PART THREE

After having chosen Merton and Gandhi as examples of mature spirituality, I was pleasantly surprised to find that James Fowler, in his *The Stages of Faith,* has given them as examples of the highest level of spiritual growth.

11. THOMAS MERTON

"Thomas Merton was ahead of his time on almost every front: religious renewal, the relationship of action and contemplation in the Christian life, ecumenism in the broadest terms, the importance of narrative for theology."[1] [Elena Malits]

Thomas Merton is undoubtedly one of the greatest spiritual leaders of our time. Like all great leaders, he addressed many of the important issues of his time; as a spiritual teacher, he transcended the times and addressed the eternal issues of human life. When this Catholic monk who belonged to the Trappist monastic order died in 1968, the New York Times referred to him as the best-known monk since Luther. That distinction still holds true. A man of many qualities and multiple talents, he was a poet and a philosopher, a contemplative and a *karma yogi* (spiritual activist), a committed Catholic monk and a genuine ecumenist.

Merton's Life History In Brief

Merton's fascinating life went through several stages. His childhood was unstable and lonely; his youth was rebellious; his young adulthood was one of intense search for the meaning of life; finally, he became a Catholic and later joined a Trappist monastery at age 26. His monastic life also went through many phases: blind obedience, conflicts and more independence, active participation in the socio-political issues of his time, life as a hermit, an experience of romantic love, and finally a journey to Asia during which he had a profound mystical experience.

He was born in Prades, France on January 31, 1915. His father, Owen Merton, painter and pianist, came from New Zealand; his mother, Ruth Merton, was American. They had met and married in Paris. Europe was already embroiled in World War I and according to French law Merton was subject to conscription. So they decided to move to America. Thomas Merton was only a year old when the family settled in Flushing, Long Island, just a few miles from where Ruth's parents lived. Thomas's brother, John Paul, was born in November 1918.

Ruth Merton was a versatile, ambitious, and perfectionist woman. Thomas Merton remembered her chiefly as a worried person. She had read the manuals on childcare and tried to follow them closely. 'Color' was one of the first words uttered by little Tom. After John Paul was born, Tom began to lose the total attention of his mother. He became rather rebellious, and his mother's discipline grew more harsh.

Ruth Merton had little use for organized religion. She wanted Tom to be independent and original. Her perfectionism left him with a sense of rejection, and a sense of disappointment in himself. Owen Merton was a successful painter, energetic and independent. He was also self-critical as good artists often are. He had a deep faith based on the doctrines of the Church of England. While living in Flushing, he attended Quaker meetings and took Tom with him at times.

Tom was a lonely child because John Paul was too young to play with and there were no children of Tom's age in the neighborhood. So he invented an imaginary friend named Jack and an imaginary dog called Doolittle. One time Tom refused to cross a street for fear that Doolittle might get run over by a car.

When Tom was only six years old, his mother was hospitalized with stomach cancer. She wanted Tom to grow up as an optimistic, strong person, so she didn't want him to visit her and be exposed to sickness and death. One day she sent a note through Owen informing Tom that she was dying. This caused Tom a heavy burden of sadness. Years later, he expressed how nice it would have been if he had known how to pray then. When his mother passed away, Tom was not allowed to visit her or attend the cremation.

After their mother's death, Tom and John Paul lived with their grandparents for a while. Then Owen Merton took Tom with him on his painting trips. The father and son developed a special intimacy during those days. Owen had become more spiritually active since his wife's death. He tried to get his son interested in religion. For a while they lived in France and Tom was impressed by a couple, the Privats, with whom they stayed for a while. The Privats were a devoutly Catholic couple—simple, loving, and kind farmers. After France, Tom and his father moved to England.

In England Tom went to school at Oakham. He involved himself enthusiastically in his studies and extracurricular activities. He was very sociable and had many friends. He did not show off the superior knowledge acquired from his wide reading and travels.

The school Chaplain equated the English idea of gentlemanliness with Christianity. Tom could see through the superficial, but he did not point a finger at others. At that time, the British were finding an unprecedented critic of their way of life and beliefs in a man named Gandhi. The young friends of Merton made fun of the little brown man (as youngsters often do) who was challenging the mighty Empire. Merton saw Gandhi in a different light and wrote a paper in support of him. That displeased his colleagues, but did not daunt Merton.

In 1929 Owen Merton became ill and was admitted to a hospital in London. He died of a brain tumor the following year. Upon visiting his father in the hospital, Tom had noticed his father's deep religious faith even in the midst of suffering. Tom had a hunch that his father was using his suffering to transform himself spiritually to reach God. Following Owen Merton's death, his friend Dr. Bennett became Tom's guardian. From the Bennetts, Tom learned about Hemingway, D. H. Lawrence, Gide, and Blake. Too late, he learned that the writings of D. H. Lawrence and others were meant for esthetic enjoyment and not for moral guidelines.

He went on a vacation to Italy before entering Cambridge. In Italy he became more interested in Christianity. One night he had a religious experience while alone in his room with the lights on. Suddenly he experienced the presence of his father in the room. The father's-presence experience passed in a flash but the event left him with an overwhelming sense of inner corruption and an intense desire for liberation from it. He began to pray from the depth of his heart. However, much more corruption and confusion would befall him before his final change.

Then came a year at Cambridge—his time of 'acting out'. He indulged in drinking and sex; he cut lectures and even got arrested one time for a traffic violation. He made a girl pregnant. Besides these experiences, an acquaintance committed suicide by hanging himself in the showers.

Dr. Bennett had enough troubles and was glad to let Merton return to America. It is believed that Dr. Bennett settled matters with the parents of the girl whom Merton had made pregnant. Apparently the mother and child were killed in the German air raids on London.

Merton entered Columbia University in 1935, where Professor Mark Van Doren, who taught English Literature, had a remarkable influence on him. Van Doren's objectivity, honesty, and love of his subject were impressive. Blake and Dante stimulated Merton's interest in Catholicism. Blake was a staunch critic of the false piety that replaced charity and love of God with formalisms and formulas. Merton also had some exposure to Communist ideology. He became very close to his maternal grandfather, but the latter died the following year.

A friend introduced Merton to Bramachari, a Hindu monk whose simplicity, sense of humor, openness, and compassion impressed Merton. Interestingly, Bramachari recommended that Merton read *The Imitation of Christ* and St. Augustine's *Confessions*. These and other influences (such as further interest in Blake and the writings of Jacques Maritain) nudged him toward Catholicism. After the long search, Merton became a Catholic. With the characteristic energy and commitment to whatever he did, Merton did not settle for being a lay Catholic but wanted to become a priest and, even more, a monk.

He tried to join the Franciscans, but after a few months he had the urge to confess his past misadventures to them. It was really unnecessary for him to do so because those sins had been confessed and absolved before. Once he disclosed the secrets, the Franciscans rejected him. Adding insult to injury, a Capuchin friar to whom he confessed misunderstood him and chided him further.

Later he became interested in joining the Trappist monks and they accepted him, knowing all his background. He entered the Trappist monastery at Gethsemani near Louisville, Kentucky in December 1941. The monks practiced silence, simple vegetarian diets, short hours of sleep, long hours of prayer, strict obedience, and hard physical labor on the farm of the monastery. Merton followed all these enthusiastically. He enjoyed the nearness to nature. He had finally found a home, and that meant much to a person who lost both parents early in life. Even the last remaining member of his immediate family, his brother John Paul, died in 1943 in a plane crash. A few months before, John Paul had visited Merton in the monastery and had joined the Catholic Church.

At Gethsemani his long loneliness was transformed into solitude. Even in the middle of a busy monastic life he found time to write. He made translations from French and Latin and produced some pamphlets for the Trappists. His abbot recognized Merton's talent, and gave him the freedom to pursue his writing. Merton's first major work was his autobiographical *The Seven Storey Mountain*. His book was a big success—it sold 100,000 copies by the time he was ordained a priest in May 1949.

In 1948 Dom James Fox, a graduate of Harvard Business School, took over as abbot. James Fox and Merton had some conflicts; Fox was more authoritarian than his predecessor. Despite differences of opinion, James Fox had great respect for Merton and indeed chose him to be his personal confessor. Their conflict had reached a point where Merton had even tried to join another order. Finally Merton's request to become the novice master was granted and his ability to nurture spiritual growth in others found a good outlet. He detested dishonesty and emphaized authenticity. His pupils loved and respected him. They also appreciated his sharp sense of humor.

In the 1950's Merton continued to become more independent; he gradually gained more freedom to pursue his writing. And in the 1960's Merton became increasingly involved in the socio-political issues of the world. He was a voracious reader and a prolific writer. He read widely in psychology, sociology, literature, philosophy, and of course religion. In religion, besides Christianity, he learned more about Buddhism, Judaism, Taoism, Sufism, and Hinduism. His knowledge of these varied subjects was deep and genuine and it

difffered completely from that of religious fanatics who learn some of
the weak points of particular religions so that they can look down on
the faiths of others and strut sickly proud of their own. Merton's
writings clearly show the depth of his understanding of various fields,
reflecting his objectivity and great capacity for empathy.

Merton wrote literary essays, poems and books, and he wrote
extensively on various aspects of religious and social issues. From the
perspective of a contemplative who was keenly aware of the needs
and weaknesses of human beings, he expressed his ideas about
spiritual and social issues in ways that touched peoples' hearts and
minds. He corresponded with hundreds of people.

Merton wrote about love and hate, war and non-violence, racial
discrimination and the need for understanding. He was an admirer of
Gandhi and understood Gandhi's ideas of non-violence more deeply
and clearly than most people. In his writings, when he discusses the
ideas of psychoanalyst Erich Fromm, Zen Master D. T. Suzuki, or
Taoist Chaung Tzu, it is clear that Merton had well digested,
absorbed, and internalized their ideas.

Merton worked for ecumenism and East-West understanding; he
worked against the Viet Nam War and and the Nuclear Arms Race.
These activities made him a friend of many and a foe of many others.
There were death threats against him. Church hierarchy brought
pressure to stop him from publishing anti-war letters and articles.
However, he was permitted to send out mimeographed copies and he
did that. Some of his close friends helped him with this somewhat
"bootleg" operation.

In the last decade of his life Merton had several health problems
including bursitis and colitis. He carried an enormous work load for
years. Besides other doctors, he also consulted a psychiatrist. The
psychiatrist found that Merton not only was not neurotic, but
psychologically strong.

For a long time Merton had wanted to live in a hermitage; he
finally received permission in 1963. He enjoyed the solitude of
hermitage life and living close to nature. It reduced his stresses and he
could sleep better. He did not isolate himself too much but joined his
fellow monks for Mass and continued his work with novices.

In March 1966, he underwent surgery for cervical spondylosis.
While recovering, he fell in love with a student nurse half his age. It
was a passionate and mutual love. For six months he poured out his
heart in poetry and letters, phone calls, and sometimes contrived
visits. He made use of some of his friends to help him in the visits, but
they often refused to cooperate. His relationship finally came to an
end after confessing to his spiritual director and abiding by his
recommendations. Merton, who had felt a sense of rejection from his
mother and had gotten into hot water with his youthful sexuality,

had gradually developed an ease and trust in his relationship with women long before he fell in love with this pretty and energetic nurse. His biographer Michael Mott notes that this love was an overwhelming experience for Merton; it brought on a permanent change. It cleared any doubts he had of his ability to love or to be loved. "Thomas Merton had found his authentic wholeness in authentic love."[2]

He had long wanted to visit Asia and a very good occasion came up—a conference of monastic leaders of various religions to be held at Bangkok during December 1968. He visited several places in India and Sri Lanka before he got to Bangkok for the conference. During his visits he met several religious leaders, including the Dalai Lama. Merton found the Dalai Lama open-minded even about Marxism in spite of the sufferings of Tibetan Buddhists under the rule of Chinese Communists. The Dalai Lama admired Merton's open-mindedness, depth of understanding, and sincerity.

At Polonnaruwa in Sri Lanka he visited the huge Buddha statues carved out from rocks. His companion, the Vicar General of the local diocese, kept away from the "pagan" place. Merton approached the Buddhas barefoot. The great smiles, the peace and sense of acceptance impressed Merton greatly. Never before had he found such a "sense of beauty and spiritual validity running together in one aesthetic illumination."[3] He had a sense of having penetrated the surface, gone beyond the shadow and seen what he was looking for. James Laughlin, a long-time friend of Merton, remarks how appropriate it was that Merton had his great mystical experience through his ecumenism.[4] A friend of mine observed that it was God's way of affirming the validity of genuine ecumenism. Also remarkable is what the formalistic Vicar Generals of this world miss.

On December 10, 1968 Merton spoke on "Marxism and monastic prespective." He noted how both the monk and the Marxist are aiming at change. While the Marxist tries for external or social change, the monk works for internal change or change of consciousness. The essence of monastic life is a transformation from selfish love to genuine love. There was some of the same desire in Marx. Merton also talked about the idea of alienation, a basically Christian idea which was given importance by Marx and more recently by Erich Fromm. He concluded with a call for interdependence and inner transformation.

After the speech he had lunch and then he went off to his room. That afternoon, he was accidentally electrocuted and died alone in his room. It was on the 27th anniversary of his entering the monastery. Born during the first winter of the First World War, he died in the shadow of the Viet Nam War. Ironically, the dead body of this man of peace was brought to the United States for burial by an Air Force plane.

Elements of Mature Spirituality in Merton

Courage and Prudence—It take tremendous courage to be open minded, to let oneself be vulnerable to various world views as Merton did. He was searching openly forever for deeper and wider knowledge. He was not looking for additional support for a narrow world view he had chosen once and for all.

In order to transcend narcissistic and egoistic tendencies and to love genuinely, one has to take the risks of potential rejection or hurt. Merton was a loving soul not just to family and friends but to all. It took a lot of courage to be so loving. He even dared to fall in love in his fifties.

Creative work requires a good deal of courage. As he grew older and wiser, Merton showed more daring in his writings, as well as in other aspects of his life. In the words of Deba Patnaik, a poet and friend of Merton, "As Merton evolved from his earlier poetry of traditional diction, meter and symbolist preoccupation, he displayed a remarkable consummation of his life and art, of daring experimentation."[5]

In pursuing his twin vocations—as a contemplative and as a writer—Merton showed the courage to be the person he really was. He did not let one aspect suppress the other.

Merton showed great prudence or caution in the important matters of his life, as in his momentous decision to become a monk. For the monastic life provided the discipline, the peace and quiet, the solitude, and the distance from the distracting world, all of which nurtured the best in him to become a great monk and a great writer. Had his choice of life style been less prudent, his energies could have been wasted or even channeled into destructive activities. He showed his caution in keeping to his commitments and following the directions of his spiritual guide and his other authorities. He accepted the censoring of his anti-war letters by church officials. He ended his romantic love with the student nurse at the direction of his spiritual guide. He took great pains to prevent hurting others. He had the prudence to seek help when he needed it, including psychiatric consultation when he was under heavy stress.

Love—Merton was loving toward everyone: his friends, the novices he taught, the people he corresponded with, all attest his nurturing nature. His writings clearly reflect his deep love for everyone and his compassion for the underdogs. Genuine love, not personal ambition, involved him in the socio-political issues. In fact, he could have had much more acclaim from many powerful circles if he had avoided social activism. He called the Vietnamese Buddhist leader, Naht Hanh, his brother. His falling in love also shows that he had neither killed his passions nor let them degenerate into masochism or hate of others. He had only transformed his passions into the fruits of love.

Therefore, at a time of stress and regression, the passion could sprout.

Merton had a healthy self-esteem without which he could not have handled the many big losses of his life as well as he did. He did not try to negate the fact that he was a famous author. He was humble but he did not humiliate himself.

As for love of God, is there any question that this passionate and intelligent man's dedication to monastic life was ultimately because of his love of God? Love of God is a central theme in many of his writings. His enthusiasm for non-violence was also rooted in his love of God and love of all beings, all creatures of God.

Merton did not keep grudges or nurse grievances. Even his conflicts with Dom James Fox did not turn into hate. There is no hint of hate in his autobiographical writings about people who had hurt him. John Eudes Bamberger, Merton's physician and fellow monk, has stated that he never noticed bitterness in Merton.

What religious people often hate are other religions and Communism. Merton is a well-known exception to this rule. He could see the differences and similarities in other world views. He did not love every aspect of every religion or ideology. He warned people against uncritical adoption of Zen or other religious practices. He consistently liked the spiritually healthy aspects of religion. It is the mystical aspect of other religions that often appealed to him most. When he spoke of Communism, it is the ideas against alienation and in favor of brotherly love that Merton commended; he was not supporting many other aspects of Communism.

Merton did not show narcissism and egoism. His great success as a writer did not go to his head; nor did the money go to his pocket. Greed had no place in his life. He could see very clearly the mess the wise moderns were creating because of greed. He had no conflict with the simplicity of monastic life although he had conflicts with excessive obedience. He fought against the group narcissism and the group egoism of his religion, nation, and race.

Merton made many profound observations on love. I will quote just a few here from the book *Love and Living*:

> "Love is, in fact, an intensification of life, a completeness, a fullness, a wholeness of life."[6]

> "We do not become fully human until we give ourselves to each other in love."[7]

> "Love is our true destiny."[8]

> "We will never be fully real until we let ourselves fall in love—either with another human person or with god."[9] (Evidently Merton did both).

"Genuine love is a personal revolution."[10]

"Love is not a deal, it is a sacrifice. It is not marketing, it is a form of worship."[11]

Wisdom

We saw that he was open to various schools of thought. He was a person deeply committed to his own faith but he did not close his mind around the dogmas of his Church. He was always curious, always searching and learning. However, he was not addicted to or even interested in collecting trivia. His intellectual energy was spent on learning and understanding mattters of deep concern spiritually, socially, and psychologically. If he appeals to intellectuals of various hues, this is the main reason.

Wisdom lies in good discerment, and for that, one has to have good insight into one's strengths and weaknesses and an understanding of the meaning of life. Healthy insight makes us aware of our limitations. Even much later in his life, when he needed the help of another authority, he accepted it. The depth of his insight is evident in all his writings. Indeed, it is his wisdom that enabled him to understand other people's points of view so well. He could easily have settled down with the idea "I found it" when he became a Catholic or a Trappist. But he did not.

His deep interest in the mystical writings of Meister Eckhart—the 14th Century monk and mystic who was posthumously condemned by the Pope—and in other religions, particularly Buddhism, played a major role in Merton's spiritual growth. Mathew Fox, a Catholic monk and scholar on Eckhart, observes: "Merton confesses to having been 'entranced' by Meister Eckhart, and it can be documented that his conversion from being a romantic dualistic and Augustinian-minded monk in the fifties to being a prophetic Christian in the sixties occurred while he was studying Zen and Meister Eckhart."[12]

Highly Integrated Personality—In his writings he staunchly opposed compartmentalization. He also denounced alienation. His action, his beliefs, and the ideas he expressed in his writings were all consistent. The depth of his spirituality pervaded everything about him. He used the mature psychological defenses of humor, altruism, suppression, anticipation, and sublimation. He had faced the major existential dilemmas squarely. His spirituality, combining solitude and spiritual activism with genuine compassion and love for all, was his answer to the existential questions. His contemplative life and creative work provided the deep meaning in his life.

Merton was open and honest about his follies and foibles. Unlike many people with fame, he did not try to keep up an 'image'. As he advanced spiritually, he revised his opinions and expressed them honestly. Monica Furlong, a biographer of Merton, noted how he had treated Oriental mysticism with a sense of Catholic superiority in *The Seven Storey Mountain*.[13] Later he learned more about Eastern mysticism, his opinions changed, and in his *Asian Journal* he admitted that he found deep spiritual attainment and certitude in eastern mystics. What may appear to superficial observers as inconsistency was really a deeper consistency and integration.

Suprisingly for all the instability of his childhood, Merton showed a healthy holistic identity. He did not discriminate or exclude anybody on the basis of religion, class, race, ethnic background, and the like. Indeed, as a mystic he realized his true identity in the depth of his being and its connectedness to the Ultimate Being. As a man he was neither a macho nor a wimp, but a holistic person integrating masculine strength and femine tenderness. He was not ashamed of his sensitiveness.

In my conversations with Trappist monks, I was impressed by their admiration for Merton as a well integrated person. One of them, a student of Merton, put it beautifully: "Merton is the most integrated, most well-put-together person I have known." Merton was well disciplined. Even as he was working on many books and had interesting ideas to talk about, Merton's lectures were focused on the assigned topic, not distracted by his personal interests. Merton's lectures contained a good sense of humor but it was not artificial; it came with the natural flow of his talks.

His enthusiasm was strong, making his lectures very attractive. He spent a few minutes of his lecture just talking about some simple incident that happened to him such as a bird that flew overhead as he was walking that day. This approach helped his students to get better grounded in the here and now. That way they could better connect the theoretical concepts and the everyday world of reality.

Merton's strong sense of humor was something that people around him enjoyed a lot. Although his writings are often serious, one can notice sense of humor in between. At one place he talked about sin being quite different from making an ass of oneself. In *My Argument With the Gestapo* the poet-hero is interrogated by the French police about his private journal. The interrogation is hilarious because of the assumption by the police that anything written is of a political nature. Another person who knew that the journal was neither pro-British nor pro-German thought it must be pornographic. Joan Baez has said that during the time she spent with Merton they mostly laughed.

His life as a monk and social activist clearly illustrated sublimation and altruism. Merton was fascinated by the ideas of alienation and by the ideas of final integration elaborated by Arestah and others. Merton's special interest in these ideas reflect his own final integration and his keen awareness of the forces of alienation in society and in his own past.

He loved simplicity; the monastic life provided it easily. He needed solitude; the hermitage provided it well. However, he enjoyed the simple pleasures of life including drinking a beer now and then. Although he had strong discipline and strong will, he was willing to surrender to the greater mystery of life. Therefore he gained more intuitive wisdom and he had mystical (peak) experiences.

Along with and beyond his simplicity Merton had tremendous depth. The depth of his interests was clearly reflected in the penetrating understanding he developed on the broad spectrum of psychological, spiritual, and social issues that really mattered. He was prophetic in his vision of the dangers of the nuclear arms race and the need for a better understanding between different religions and ideologies. He foresaw the tragic course of the Vietnam War and the racial conflicts in the U.S. before most others did.

The continuing popularity of Merton is an indication of the attraction people have toward authentic spirituality and integrated personality. The religious people who deplore the dearth of spirituality in modern times might well take a serious look at this fact, and examine whether their own house is in order. The last decade of Merton's life was a fitting answer to the crucial question Nietzsche had posed long ago, "If Christians wish us to believe in their Redeemer, why don't they look a little more redeemed?" If he were alive today, Nietzsche, who claimed that the last Christian died on the cross, might pose another question, "If religion has wisdom, why doesn't it produce more integrated people like Merton?"

12.   MAHATMA   GANDHI

"It is certainly true that Gandhi was not above all criticism; no man is. But it is evident that he was unlike all the other world leaders of his time in that his life was marked by a wholeness and a wisdom, an integrity others lacked, or manifested only in reverse, in consistent fidelity to a dynamism of evil and destruction."[1] [Thomas Merton]

Mohandas K. Gandhi, who came to be known as Mahatma (great soul) Gandhi, was born in October 2, 1869 in Porbandar in Western India. His father had worked as Prime Minister of the local King. The family were devout Hindus, particularly Gandhi's mother, who lived a simple and pious life.

He was not especially remarkable as a child. As a schoolboy he was not bright, but he was punctual. He was shy and introverted— characteristics often considered undesirable. But they made him sensitive to others and careful in his speech and action. Gandhi described his shyness as his shield.

At the tender age of thirteen, he married the girl his parents had picked for him according to the custom of the day. He was a domineering and insecure husband. Gandhi's sense of inferiority vis-a-vis his wife was based on his fears about thieves, snakes, ghosts, and the like, which did not bother his wife. She was illiterate and had no interest in studies. Gandhi's attempts at educating his young wife and making her his intellectual companion failed. Therefore Gandhi had to settle for the role of a traditional husband.

He had his share of youthful follies and foibles. He and a relative experimented with smoking, and he stole some coins from the servants of the family for that purpose. They could not smoke in the presence of elders. This lack of freedom led them to such despair that they decided to commit suicide. They collected Dhatura seeds, which are poisonous, and went to the temple with the intention of swallowing the seeds and dying there. However, when the moment came, they had second thoughts; and they changed their minds. The thought of suicide changed them—they quit smoking and stealing pennies from the servants. As Nietzsche observed, one takes life seriously after contemplating suicide.

Thin and nonathletic himself, Gandhi was envious of the strong and athletic boys. One such boy attributed his strength to the habit of meat eating. So, Gandhi tried to strengthen himself by eating meat, against the belief of his parents. He had to do it surreptitiously. Gradually he decided that he would rather settle for being weak than being dishonest, and he quit eating meat.

Gandhi's friend took him to a brothel once and made all the arrangements. When the time came, Gandhi just sat near the woman on the bed and made no further moves. The woman slowly lost her cool and, with insults, got him out of the house. Gandhi's description of these incidents shows truthfulness, a gentle sense of humor, and a deep acceptance of himself. There is no evidence of self-hate or wallowing in guilt. His openness and eagerness to make amends and his resoluteness were remarkable.

The incident, at age fifteen, of stealing a bit of gold from his brother is particularly touching. He felt guilty and resolved never to steal again. Gandhi was not afraid of punishment from his father, but he was concerned about hurting his father's feelings. Gandhi wrote his confession on a paper and gave it to his ailing father. His father shed tears as he sat up and read it, then lay back down. Gandhi also cried. Nothing was said, and yet there was deep communication of total understanding and deep love. It was a lesson in nonviolence for Gandhi—an experience of inner transformation and relating to others with that inner harmony.

His father passed away when Gandhi was sixteen. Gandhi had nursed his father devotedly during the years the latter was sick. This nurturing quality blossomed later into the nurturing of a whole country and, in that process, the nurturing of a large part of humanity that was in the grip of destructive forces.

As a youngster, he didn't care much for religion, but he listened to discussions at home by devotees of Hinduism, Jainism, and Islam about their different viewpoints. This early exposure to different religions must have helped him to be quite open minded. In the film *Gandhi*, there are some beautiful and highly relevant flashbacks of Gandhi's childhood. One of these shows Gandhi tellng an American journalist that the priest in his temple used to read from Hindu scripture Bhagavad Gita and from Moslem's Koran. Thus he was exposed to genuine ecumenism.

During the nearly three years he spent in England studying law, he was preoccupied with personal and moral issues as well. Before leaving for England, he made a vow that he would not touch meat, wine, or women, and that had relieved his anxious mother. He kept his vows strictly. Later in life he realized that making a vow opened up real freedom rather than closing it up. That helped him to make strong commitments.

Gandhi's experience with Christianity in India was quite negative. He was exposed to the speeches of Christian missionaries who were contemptuous and ignorant of Hindus and their gods. He had also heard of people who were converted to Christianity who had to eat beef, drink liquor, and wear European clothes. All these negative impressions still did not make him close his mind against

Christianity. Therefore, while in England, he became interested in learning more about Christianity. When he read the book of Genesis and the book of Numbers, they bored him; but he persisted. The Sermon on the Mount caught his imagination. The message of the Beatitudes became an integral part of his philosophy of life.

Here we can see some important characteristics of the mahatma that made him a unique spiritual leader—his openness in spite of negative experiences and his acceptance of the good parts of something even if he didn't care for some other of its aspects. Gandhi's attraction to the Sermon on the Mount also illustrated his keen eye for the essence of a religion or an idelogy. Away from home and country, he also became more interested in Hinduism, especially in BhagavadGita, which Gandhi called his spiritual reference book. Gandhi's ideal of man was largely based on the teachings of this holy book. That ideal involves lack of egotism and selfishness, dedication to truth and commitment to action, using fair means on the basis of truth, without focusing on the end result. Gandhi noted that those who focus on the end result rather than the process may lose their nerve in performing their duty, or may use improper means to achieve the end.

The problem of focusing on an end result is encountered often in psychiatric disorders. One typical example is sexual dysfunctions where the fear of performance failure perpetuates the problem in people who are focusing on orgasm rather than enjoying the process of sexual union. Detachment from the results does not mean lack of direction and purpose in the action. The direction and purpose are certainly imbedded in the choice of action which is to be made in accordance with truth and duty. There is certainly great psychological merit in this approach.

Gandhi met many earnest men and women in England who were opposed to the Victorian Establishment—people who believed in simple living and high thinking. He also read widely. Tolstoy's *The Kingdom of God is Within You* had great influence on Gandhi. So, also, did Ruskin's *Unto This Last*. Upon his return to India, Gandhi was deeply influenced by a third writer, the poet Raychard. Emerson and Thoreau also impressed him.

When he returned to India, he was shocked to find that his mother had passed away. Other shocks were awaiting him. He found out that it was not easy to establish himself as a lawyer. His shyness made him unable to plead his case in court. However, because of family influence he was able to set up an office practice drafting applications and memorials. Then he got a job in South Africa.

In South Africa, Gandhi experienced extreme racial discrimination. Once when he was traveling in first class he was thrown off the train because he refused to travel in third class, meant for colored people. This was Gandhi's moment of truth. He could either put up with such injustice, go back to India, or stay and fight against it. He chose to stay and fight against the injustices. Whether or nor Sartre's argument holds good in general—that when an individual makes an important choice for himself/herself, he/she is making a choice for the whole of humanity—here was an instance where it was dramatically true.

The courage of his convictions about the truth of his cause transformed the shy, retiring Gandhi into an able political leader almost over night. The man who went to South Africa to work as a lawyer became a political leader of the Indian community and lived there 21 years. Those were long, hard years of struggle against great odds—years that further solidified Gandhi's political and spiritual ideals and techniques. He believed in Satyagraha (firmness in truth) as the appropriate method to bring about change. Following this ideology, he and his followers resisted unjust laws by civil disobedience, protest marches, and willingness to be imprisoned. About two years after going to South Africa, Gandhi went back to India to take his wife and children with him. He and his wife, Kasturbai, had conflicts over his ideals of equality of all races and castes. His orthodox wife was unhappy about having a former untouchable as a boarder in their house. The couple had a shouting match over it and then both changed for the better—Kasturbai became more tolerant and Gandhi learned to control his temper. Gandhi admitted that he learned a great deal of love and patience from his wife.

An incident early in his career in South Africa illustrates Gandhi's difference as a lawyer. Attorneys in general thrive on adversarial approaches. In a 1967 film *Divorce American Style*, a couple, having minor marital conflicts, consulted their lawyers. As the husband and wife followed the recommendations of their respective attorneys, the couple's marital problems mushroomed into major issues and ended in a bitter divorce. Such are too often the consequences of an adversarial approach. Gandhi had a client named Dada Abdulla who had legal problems with a relative. If the conflict went on for long, as it would have with the usual process, Abdulla and his relative would have lost more money and the conflict between the men and their families would have gotten worse. Gandhi worked very hard with his client and the opponent to settle the matter out of court. It meant losing a lot of potential income for Gandhi. In the end, Abdulla and his opponent were quite happy. Gandhi gained more insight into the process of negotiation and cooperative-creative relating. According to Gandhi, the true function of an attorney is to unite the opponents.

In the struggle against the unjust rules of South African government, hundreds of Indian men and women actively participated. They went to jail, were subjected to floggings, struck work, and even faced being shot. Gandhi himself was in jail several times. Finally in June 1914, Gandhi and the South African leader, Smuts, reached an agreement. According to the agreement, Hindu, Moslem, and Parsi marriages, and not just Christian marriages, were considered valid. A three pound tax on indentured laborers was canceled, and free Indians (not indentured laborers) could continue to enter South Africa.

There were two interesting incidents during the struggle. One was that Gandhi formed an Indian Ambulance corps and helped the wounded British soldiers in the war against Dutch soldiers. He was awarded the War Medal by the British. During an uprising of the Zulu tribe, Gandhi's ambulance aided wounded British soldiers and natives. These facts have been distorted in anti-Gandhi propaganda to make Gandhi appear a warmonger during that part of his life. Gandhi did not hate the British or anyone else whom he opposed. Moreover, his idea was to modify the system and stay within the British Empire. It was only years later, after seeing the terrible damage that British rule was doing to India, that Gandhi wanted the British rule to end. If this shows a lack of hot nationalism, it also shows the far greater human qualities of openness, the search for compromise, willingness to understand, tolerance and, above all, a holistic identity.

The other interesting incident was that Gandhi made a pair of sandals for his opponent, Smuts, when Gandhi was in jail. This act was undertaken in genuine good spirits and Smuts took it at face value. Smuts had great respect for Gandhi. Gandhi practiced what he preached about working to change the heart of the enemy. Those who believe in extreme dualism see the only possibility of dealing with enemies as isolating and destroying them, or isolating oneself.

A grateful Indian community in South Africa had given many presents to Gandhi, but he was distressed about it. He did not want to keep the gifts or use them because that would go against his desire for selfless service. He did not want to reject the gifts because it would hurt the feelings of the people who were dear to him. So, he created a trust and put the gifts into the trust to be used for community service.

Gandhi returned to India for good in 1915. He soon became leader of the freedom movement which was already gathering momentum. On both the Indian side and the British side there were people who believed in the use of force, and others who believed in negotiated changes. An Indian historian told Gandhi that nonviolence had never freed a country, but Gandhi pointed out that one important lesson in history is that unprecedented events do happen. Gandhi, and under his influence the vast majority of his party, the Indian National Congress, believed in nonviolent change. Officialdom in

England often seemed to believe in the age-old military formula about opponents—"force is the only thing they respect."

When the wartime restrictions were continued by the British after the war, Gandhi called for civil disobedience and peaceful protests. Against Gandhi's instructions and wishes, violence broke out in different parts of the country. Gandhi called off the campaign, admitted it was a big mistake, and fasted for three days as penance. Gandhi's willingness to admit mistakes and change a course of action was a rare quality for a politician. In fact, the Viceroy is said to have admitted that he was scared to meet with Gandhi because Gandhi could admit mistakes and change a course of action whereas the Viceroy could not do the same.

During the above-mentioned campaign, a British officer ordered his forces to shoot at unarmed civilians at a peaceful meeting in Amritsar, killing 379 people and injuring 1,137. This officer wanted to teach the Indians a lesson. The result of that massacre was renewed determination by Indians to get the colonialists out. Gandhi launched a movement of non-cooperation. When the King announced some reforms, Gandhi called off the non-cooperation movement, again showing his belief in cooperation rather than confrontation.

Gandhi was fighting several evils at the same time. British colonialism was only one of those. That itself would have been a simpler task except for the other complex problems he had to tackle: the system of untouchability, Hindu-Moslem conflicts, slavish mentality, and divisive tendencies.

The struggle with the British Empire was not an easy one as some people in the West seem to conceive. The British government, especially under Churchill, had no intention of giving Indians political freedom, or even much lesser rights. Gandhi spent years in jail. In March 1922, he was tried in the court of law on charges of exciting disaffection against his Majesty's government. Gandhi's brilliant defense of himself really put the colonial justice system itself on trial. Gandhi pointed out that the law in British India was intended to exploit the masses. He blamed both the Englishmen and their Indian associates for perpetuating the crime. Everyone is obliged to cooperate with good but not with evil, he asserted. On this occasion he was sentenced to six years imprisonment; on many other occasions he was imprisoned without a trial. His wife died in 1944 while she was imprisoned with him.

Untouchability had become a well-entrenched system of severe discrimination against the lowest strata of society. To change such an age-old system was an enormously difficult job. And of course, Gandhi did it in his nonviolent way—changing the hearts of the victimizers and the victims. He brought it about through speeches and writings, prayer meetings, and above all by personal example. Hindu-Moslem animosity had to be tackled delicately. Gandhi attempted it in the same way as with other struggles—with love. He knew both sides of the issue well and helped others to know. His respect for all religions, not mere tolerance, set the example. He showed his sincere caring for people of all religions, and he responded to the needs of Moslems to feel secure in a country of overwhelming Hindu majority.

Nearly two centuries of foreign exploitation saw the decline of India from one of the richest regions of the world to one of the poorest. Along with the material poverty, there were also the poor self-esteem, excessive fears, and unhealthy rigidities. Gandhi's brilliance lay in transforming the millions from a state of inferiority complex to a state of self-affirmation without going overboard into a superiority complex.

Gandhi's attempts to reconcile Hindus and Moslems was the most difficult problem he faced. Ultimately his attempts failed in that Pakistan was created alongside a free India in 1947, and hundreds of thousands of people of both faiths were killed and injured in the communal clashes. Even then, Gandhi was a tremendous influence in reducing the damage. The uncompromising opposition of Jinnah— the Moslem leader who was the opposite of Gandhi in most respects—was a major cause of Gandhi's failure to achieve Hindu-Moslem unity. Until his death Gandhi continued to work for a better relationship between the two communities.

When he was not in jail, Gandhi lived most of the time in what is called ashram, the spiritual commune where he and some of his ardent followers lived an exemplary village life. The life in the ashram showed how his spirit of simplicity, discipline, cleanliness, love, and search for truth can be practiced in the every-day world. The huts of the ashram were made with mud and bamboo. Gandhi and his followers in the ashram kept a simple vegetarian diet which was nutritionally sound. They had communal latrines which were kept clean. This was an important example of cleanliness to the ignorant villagers. The ashramites did not waste anything—even human and animal excreta were used to make compost and fertilize the agricultural land. All members of the ashram spent time daily in prayer, meditation, and work. They wore simple handmade clothes. In their spiritual readings they used the scriptures of various religions. Whenever possible, they used nature cures for illnesses, depending on Western medicine only when necessary. The proof of the pudding was that they were a healthy and happy household.

James Michaels, editor of *Forbes Magazine,* who was a correspondent for United Press in New Delhi in 1948, wrote about his experience of Gandhi's fast unto death. The fast occurred in January,

1948, and lasted six days. In those few days a "moral miracle" took place. The militantly anti-Moslem mood of the majority of Hindus and Sikhs gradually changed. Demonstrations against Gandhi faded and marches in his support increased. Finally even the extremists surrendered. Michaels wrote, "Had I not seen this physical demonstration of love overcoming hate, I would not have believed it. I was deeply moved. Previously a skeptic about Gandhi-ism, I became an admirer—and more than an admirer."[2]

In January, 1948, Gandhi asked the government leaders of India to pay about 125 million dollars to Pakistan as its share of the assets of India before the partition. The government leaders, Gandhi's own disciples, first refused but changed their minds and accepted the Mahatma's advice. What changed their minds was Gandhi's reaction to their argument against paying the amount—he burst into tears. I believe Gandhi's tears were not the manipulative tears of a self-centered person, nor the crocodile tears of a hypocrite, but the expression of deep sorrow at the failure of his followers to see the truth of the situation. The government leaders behaved promptly like the children responding to a mother's unselfish tears in a typical Indian family.

On January 30, 1948, Gandhi was assassinated by Nathuram Godse, who accused Gandhi of betraying Hinduism by his support of Moslems. Godse claimed Gandhi would have destroyed the Hindu nation. He and his closest accomplice received capital punishment the following year.

The last British Viceroy to India, Mountbatten, said, "Mahatma Gandhi will go down in history on a par with Buddha and Jesus Christ." How many times in history has the leader of the defeated party in an intense political struggle paid such compliments? In summing up their impression of the Mahatma, William Shirer in *Gandhi: A Memoir* and Vincent Sheean in *Mahatma Gandhi* refers to Plato's moving words about Socrates, ". . . of all the men of his time whom I have known, he was the wisest and justest and best." Romain Rolland had described Gandhi as Christ who only lacked the Cross, and Radhakrishnan, commenting on Gandhi's martyrdom, observed that we have given him the cross also.

Gandhi's Mature Spirituality

I have already given many examples of his love, courage, and wisdom. Gandhi's life—personal, social, and political—was centered and rooted in his spirituality. Indeed, he became a political leader par excellence because of the depth of his faith. Gandhian techniques are interesting and highly useful; however, what is far more important are the underlying dynamics. Techniques have to vary to suit the circumstances of their use and may, therefore, be temporary; the underlying motivations, however, hold good forever.

He derived wisdom, courage, and compassion from the essence of all religions. While he perceived that the basic tenets of all religions are similar, he also truthfully and courageously noted that all religions are imperfect. His life was dedicated to truth. For him mere tolerance of religions other than one's own is not enough because tolerance implies an assumption of the inferiority of other religions. Gandhi believed in positive regard for all religions. His regard for all religions was due to his genuine ecumenism; it was not at all a clever ploy on the part of an intelligent politician dealing with people of different faiths.

For Gandhi, liberation of India from foreign exploitation and from the shackles of unhealthy traditions became a religious duty. Arnold Toynbee noted that, in liberating India, Gandhi also liberated the British from the evils of colonialism. Gandhi did not believe in the compartmentalization of life into the sacred and the secular; all of life, certainly including public life, was sacred to him.

According to William Johnston, a Jesuit priest and Buddhist scholar, Gandhi is a splendid example of mysticism in action. In his brilliant book *The Inner Eye of Love,* Johnston says of Gandhi's seeking of union with God through love of fellow human beings: "This is different from a humanism which seeks only man or from a world-denying flight that seeks only God. It is a discovery of the world's highest value."[3] Gandhi's mysticism in action was characterized by devotion to truth, purity of intention, and unselfishness (or losing the ego as Johnston says).

Courage:

In modern times Gandhi is one of the best examples of the courage to be true to oneself and others, to face the fears of human existence, to be openminded, to love one's enemy, and to suffer for a great cause. And he did all these with prudence. Neither police beatings, nor years of imprisonment, not even the ever present possibility that the opponents might take his life deterred him from his dedication. Difficulties did not deter him. A prolific writer, the right-handed Gandhi wrote with his left hand when his right hand suffered from writer's cramps.

We have already seen how open-minded he was about religion. Similarly he was open to new approaches and negotiations with his opponents. He was quite open to criticisms, too. For example, his one-time secretary, Indulal Yajnik, after leaving Gandhi, wrote a book in gujarati (Gandhi's mother tongue) highly critical of the Mahatma, and asked him to write the introduction. Gandhi did it.

According to the BhagavadGita, the courageous are the ones who can forgive as we noted in Chapter 5. The Mahatma was indeed great in not holding grudges against individuals or groups who hurt him in any way. The manner in which he loved his enemies and often changed their hearts was uniquely courageous.

Eknath Easwaran gives an example of Gandhi's courage in the book *Gandhi the Man.* At a prayer meeting a cobra (a highly poisonous snake) crawled through the crowd. Gandhi noticed it and instructed people not to move. The cobra went straight to the platform where Gandhi was seated and crawled up over his thighs. Gandhi sat still, and soon the snake crawled away. As we saw earlier, Gandhi was terrified of snakes in his youth.

Courageous as he was, Gandhi was cautious, not foolhardy. Being aware of the violent tendencies of many of his followers, he had to call off peaceful protests often when they began turning violent. Sometimes he had to start satyagraha activities earlier than he had planned to prevent violence from breaking out. Gandhi also gave his opponents the courage to change.

Courage was so important for Gandhi that he said if there was no other choice but cowardice or violence, he would choose violence. The reason is that there is still hope for non-violence if the choice is for violence, whereas with the choice of cowardice there is little hope.

Love:

Gandhi claimed that love is the law of our true being. Louis Fischer, a biographer of Gandhi, writes: "Gandhi had no power to compel, punish, or reward. His power was nil, his authority was enormous. It came of love. Living with him one could see why he was loved: he loved. Not merely in isolated incidents, but day in and day out, morning, noon, and night for decades, in every act and word, he had manifested his love of individuals and of mankind."[4]

In dealing with his enemies Gandhi showed deep knowledge of their strengths and weaknesses as well as his own. That was quite different from the traditional arts of politics and, even more, of militarism which tend to exploit the weakness of the enemy and disregard other aspects. He showed care and respect towards his enemies, and he responded to their need for security and self-respect as well as to their need for a time for adjusting to changes. As much as possible, Gandhi even showed elements of deep love towards his opponents. Some people misunderstand Gandhi's appreciation of the good qualities of the British, seeing that as a weakness on his part. By his loving approach, Gandhi minimized hate and maximized the possibility of constructive engagement. And he remained lovable.

Absence of hate—self-hate or hate of others—as well as of narcissism and egoism were other pertinent features of the Mahatma. He did not show greed for power or wealth. When India gained independence, he refused any position of power for himself. He had good self-respect but no neurotic pride. He opposed group narcissism and group greed—things quite tempting to national leaders.

Gandhian techniques of fasting and peaceful protests worked on the principles of love. I had a professor of psychiatry with a special interest in suicide (as is said, every doctor has a pet disease), who used to say that Gandhi liberated India by threatening suicide. This is a total misunderstanding of the Gandhian fast.

In fasting, Gandhi was using an age-old religious ritual in a political context. The fast made the political process more sacred; it affirmed the belief that suffering can be redemptive; it showed the example of taking the burden of action on oneself rather than putting it on someone else's shoulders; it distracted his followers from their conflicts to attention on him. It is extremely important to note that Gandhi did not fast against the British or against his opponents. Moreover, only one time did he go on an indefinite fast—a fast unto death.

He fasted when his own people were doing wrong, mostly when they were becoming violent. By his fast, he stimulated the nurturing, loving instincts of his own people as against threatening his enemies. Hunger strikes against one's opponents are an entirely different and opposite approach to the Gandhian fast; the former may stimulates elements of fear and hate rather than love. Since Gandhi's time, 'satyagraha' techniques have often been misused to pursue unreasonable and selfish demands; it is really 'atyagraha' (greed), not 'satyagraha'.

Wisdom:

Gandhi used his power of reason and intuition by keeping his mind open to different points of view. Many of his techniques and solutions to varied problems came to him often intuitively. His practice of meditation aided that process tremendously. Once he had an intuitive idea, he not only used his power of reasoning, but also often experimented with the idea on himself before using it on a wide scale.

He took the best from different religions and accepted the universally good aspects of Eastern and Western cultures. He was not opposed to Western medicine and technology per se, but his emphasis was on self-reliance, simplicity, and natural approaches (using compost as fertilizer and using nature cures when possible). When he suffered from appendicitis, he underwent surgery without protest.

Gandhi's Highly Integrated Personality:

As we have seen, his thoughts, words, and deeds were consistent. In fact, he did not refer to old statements to make sure he would be consistent with them. His consistency was with the truth as he saw it at the moment.

He showed the mature psychological defenses of sublimation, altruism, anticipation, and humor. I will elaborate only on humor here because we have seen plenty of examples of the other three defenses already. His witty remarks also showed sharp insight and worked as eye-openers for his critics. He replied to Churchill's slur on him as the "half-naked fakir" by saying he would go as naked as possible. When a journalist asked him what he thought about Western civilization, Gandhi said it would be a good idea. Questioned about his plans to visit the King of England half dressed as usual, he said the King dressed enough for both. His reason for traveling third class on trains was because there was no fourth class. He once gave his address as Yeravda because he spent many years in Yeravda prison in Poona. Referring to Gandhi working for about fifteen hours a day for over thirty years, a journalist asked him when he was going to take a vacation. Gandhi replied that he was always on vacation.

The Mahatma had a universal identity. He saw the universality of both good and bad aspects of human beings—he said we are all children of One God, and we are tarred by the same brush. As a man, he combined paternal power and maternal care. Erik Erikson noted that Gandhi was one of the most maternal of all political leaders. In Erikson's words, "He [Gandhi] undoubtedly saw a kind of sublimated maternalism as part of the positive identity of a whole man, and certainly of a *homo religious*."[5] His intense awareness of himself and others made him believe in the possibility of changing the evil tendencies of people. Thomas Merton noted that people such as Hitler and Stalin built their systems on the idea that evil cannot be changed; it can only be destroyed. The Gandhian approach is the opposite. In fact, the statement that one must hate sin but not the sinner, which is attributed to Jesus by some people, was really made by Gandhi.

His creativeness and his being a man of peace need no elaboration; so also, his transcultural identity. All this does not mean he was perfect. Some individuals look for a blemish or an imperfection in a great person with the conscious or subconscious intention of denying the person's greatness. A farmer friend of mine uses a barnyard metaphor to illustrate such a tendency. He says the housefly shoots for the little spot of dirt (shit) on the hoof of one of the hind legs of the cow, completely unmindful of the milk-filled udders. There indeed are people who totally reject Jesus, citing the example of his cursing a fig tree for not bearing fruits when it was really not the fruit-bearing season.

A nurse once told me that she had heard that Buddha had "run away into the woods" to meditate and find the meaning of life, leaving a wife and newborn child. So she had no use for the old man or his teachings. She knew that Buddha's wife and child were well taken care of, and I told her his wife joined him many years later and became the first Buddhist nun. That did not matter much to this lady. One of Gandhi's imperfections was his unrealistic advocacy of celibacy apart from the procreative use of sex. However, Gandhi had always taught his followers to pursue the truth as they saw it rather than blindly follow him. Also he admitted that legitimate sexual expression is better than being obsessed with sex in attempting celibacy. Erik Erikson, who analyzed Gandhi's experiments with celibacy, brilliantly concluded, "As to the Mahatma's public private life, all we can say is that here was a man who both lived and wondered aloud, and with equal intensity and depth, about a multiformity of inclinations which other men hide and bury in strenuous consistency. At the end, great confusion can be a mark of greatness, too, especially if it results from the inescapable conflicts of existence."[6] Maslow's self-actualizing people have imperfections; so also the spiritually mature are humans, not angels.

The Mahatma clearly showed depth and discipline. However, the degree of discipline he showed is neither necessary nor practical for all. The degree of physical exercise that an Olympic athlete performs would be excessive for most. Gandhi had said, "My life is my message." The essence of his life was the persistent struggle to be well-integrated and to participate actively in life with that inner harmony. Others can follow his example within their own limits.

13. LITERARY CASES OF RELIGIOUS FANATICISM

We will examine two excellent examples of religious fanaticism from literature—the first one, the 'preacher novel' *Elmer Gantry* by Sinclair Lewis, and the second novel *With Faith and Fury* by Delos Banning McKown. Sinclair Lewis, the first American to receive the Nobel Prize for literature, was an eminent novelist and a keen social critic. Delos McKown is a professor of philosophy at Auburn University with a sharp sense of humor. Several characters in both novels show religious fanaticism but we will focus on the heroes Elmer Gantry and Manly John Plumwell respectively.

Both Elmer and Manly have many characteristics in common, but most impressive is the entirely different outcome of these two "true-believers" who followed their faith with fury. Elmer Gantry became a popular radio preacher and a powerful sociopolitical figure. Hence, the damage of his sick religiosity spread far and wide. Manly, on the other hand, murdered a professor of philosophy who challenged his beliefs, and ended up in a state hospital for the criminally insane. Obviously, Manly's evil was intense but confined to himself and his immediate surroundings. We can see these and other outcomes of fanaticism in our own everyday world.

The stories of Elmer and Manly have become all the more interesting because of the real life dramas of power struggle, illicit sex, blackmail, greed, and drug addiction among television evangelists. Rev. Jim Bakker abandoned his PTL ('Praise the Lord') TV empire reportedly to prevent the diabolical plot of Rev. Jimmy Swaggart for a hostile takeover. Bakker admitted having had a one-night stand with a former church secretary. Mrs. Bakker has been undergoing treatment for drug dependence. Rev. Oral Roberts collected $8 million by declaring that God might otherwise kill him. In a $90 million lawsuit Rev. Marvin Gorman accuses Jimmy Swaggart of conspiring to ruin his reputation by exaggerating the only incidence of adultery he committed. The lavish life styles, political ambitions, questionable fund-raising tactics, and attempts to control school text books are reminiscent of what Sinclair Lewis described.

Elmer Gantry is a brilliant novel and an insightful sociopsychological study. Lewis spent several years researching his subject matter. In that process he spent a great deal of time with clergymen, attended several churches regularly, preached from pulpits himself, and held a well publicized group called "Sinclair Lewis's Sunday School Class." This group consisted of ministers from several Christian denominations, a Catholic priest, a rabbi, and an agnostic. They discussed various important topics during their Thursday noon meetings. It is said that Lewis even got some evangelical pastors intoxicated with alcohol and got them to "spill out their guts." Lewis's reputation as a social observer was illustrated by an interesting incident. Soon after the publication of *Elmer Gantry,* H. G. Wells wrote an article on the American people based on Lewis's observations in his novels. In short, Elmer Gantry is no mere figment of imagination; he is true to life.

The book opens with the statement "Elmer Gantry was drunk," summing up the hero's character. He was intoxicated with selfishness, machoism, and power, besides alcohol in his youthful days. Religion provided him the tools to pursue these ends. We will focus on the dynamics of his sick religiosity. We will also deal briefly with a few characters other than Elmer, because it will enhance our understanding of the spiritual issues. Several social and personal influences played significant roles in Elmer's religious fanaticism. The influences of his community, his college, and his seminary shaped his unhealthy religiosity to a great extent. While he was open to unhealthy influences, he did not make good use of healthy forces to which he was exposed at times. The novel is fascinating in the brilliant exposition of the social and interpersonal dynamics of unhealthy religiosity and, to an extent, of the dynamics of healthy spirituality.

In the fall of 1902 Elmer Gantry—"Hell Cat" to his friends—was football captain of Terwillinger College, a Baptist institution in Kansas with a faculty of chiefly ex-ministers. Elmer had very little interest in scholarship, and no respect for piety; his admiration was for drunkenness and profanity. In spite of his athletic skills and good looks, he was not liked by his fellow students because he was too proud and greedy.

He had only one true friend, Jim Lefferts, a free thinker and lover of scholarship. Jim's influence made Elmer read his books and pass the exams, and Elmer relieved Jim's boredom. However, they were far apart intellectually and spiritually. Elmer swallowed ideas wholesale without processing them in the workshop of doubt and internalizing them. He was also full of prejudices. Jim was the opposite of Elmer in these respects.

As for the church, Jim had a contempt for it while Elmer was afraid of it. Growing up in rural Paris, Kansas, the fiery speeches of ministers had put the fear of the Lord into his young mind. At age eleven during his second conversion, he had signed a pledge renouncing the pleasures of drinking, dancing, profanity, and the like—a pledge to be broken time and time again. In Paris, the church was very important in people's lives because it provided music, oratory, painting, sculpture, rites of passage, and social events.

Elmer's mother, who had lost her husband early in their marriage, had found solace in the Bible and religious hymns. She urged Elmer to follow the same line. Another religious influence during his college days came from a fellow student, Eddie Fislinger, a budding evangelist. Elmer despised Eddie as a person but feared Eddie the evangelist holding a Bible which looked like the one his Sunday School teacher had used. In his Sunday School lessons, Elmer was highly impressed by the ambitious and powerful characters of the Bible such as David. As for what Elmer had gained from the church, Sinclair Lewis summed up, tongue in cheek, that it included everything except any longing for decency, compassion, and rationality.

The manner in which Elmer Gantry was 'saved' is interesting. The setting was the Annual Prayer week of the College YMCA, part of the national prayer week. State secretary of the YMCA, Judson Roberts, was the star attraction because he was once a football star. Eddie Fislinger had the vision of converting Elmer during the revival meeting. To pull all the possible strings and make sure his plan worked, Eddie had secretly telegraphed Elmer's mother to come for the meeting. Using every persuasive tactic at his disposal, certainly appealing to Elmer's masculine pride and craving for popularity, Judson tried his best to persuade Elmer to get saved. Along with that came the pleadings of his mother and the prompting of a cheering crowd. The situation was irresistible for Elmer. Eddie's conspiracy worked.

A few days later, Elmer spoke at the YMCA. Jim had given him a book by the atheist Robert Ingersoll. Elmer copied several sentences from Ingersoll on love and cleverly used them in an oration that moved his audience, none of whom knew the source of Elmer's ideas. The memory of his power to move the audience became the strongest urge for Elmer to become a preacher. Elmer lacked only the Divine 'call' to enter the seminary. Under the influence of alcohol one night, he concluded that he had the 'call'.

Elmer Gantry joined the Mizpah Theological Seminary of Northern Baptists. (Northern Baptists had split with the Southern Baptists before the Civil War on the ground that slavery was wrong according to the Bible.) The seminarians were ordained ministers after two years and they were sent to churches to hold Sunday service and Sunday School. Elmer and Frank Shallard, a fellow student, were sent to a country church. Elmer cleverly seduced the deacon's daughter Lulu in spite of Frank's warnings.

Frank was a free thinker and honest person. He had kept alive some of the rational and scientific outlook in spite of the seminary atmosphere where doubt was not just sinful but, worse, in bad taste. A faculty member, Dr. Zechlin, was an authentic scholar and closet agnostic. Frank was the only student who admired Dr. Zechlin. They confided in each other. Elmer hated this professor and finally exposed him. Dr. Zechlin was forced to retire and he died two years later. Before his death he sent thirty dimes to Elmer, obviously symbolic of the thirty silver coins for which Judas had betrayed Jesus to his enemies. Elmer did not know who had sent him the money or what it meant.

Lulu suspected she was pregnant and her infuriated father forced Elmer to agree to marry her. However, Elmer knew how to get out of tight corners by hook or crook. He arranged for Lulu and her cousin Floyd, who was interested in her, to get together. As innocent Lulu was accepting the consoling words and touch of Floyd, Elmer got Lulu's father to observe their intimacy. Elmer condemned Lulu roundly and freed himself of his responsibilities towards her. In fact, he feigned the role of an innocent victim, a ploy which he used many more times in his inglorious life.

Elmer's indiscretions slowly caught up with him. He was fired from his seminary for drinking and for arriving late at a chruch service. But he remained an ordained minster. He became a traveling salesman for a while but that was not so enjoyable as the business of religion. Then he met his ideal—a successful evangelist called Sharon Falconer. With considerable persistence he finally got Sharon to let him work with her. Sharon was a shrewd businesswoman and sensed that Elmer could be an asset. The first task Sharon assigned to Elmer was to give a talk on the monetary value of Christ in the commercial world.

Sharon had grandiose notions about herself. She thought of herself as a reincarnation of Joan of Arc and Catherine of Siena. She had visions of God and she heard His voices. Using lies, half-truths, feminine charms, and floods of tears, Sharon got her way in making huge collections. She introduced the techniques of 'thank offering', devoting one night of each program for it. She even remained single to attract more men converts.

Elmer's abilities bloomed under the favorable conditions he found with Sharon. Modeling after his college cheers, he introduced the 'Hallelujah Yell'. When the number of converts dwindled, Elmer went out and hired people to play the roles. Slowly Elmer became Sharon's assistant.

Elmer and Sharon were like two peas in a pod, as they say. They helped each other become more successful. Elmer started Sharon on the healing ministry. Although shaky at first, she caught on to it fast. She became all the more successful and confident. Her ambition continued to grow. She built a huge tabernacle, the first in a series that were planned to be built. Even in the thick of all this glamor, Elmer could not resist the opportunity to womanize. This time his attention fell on a pretty but anemic pianist. One night when he was proceeding systematically with his attempt to seduce the pianist, Sharon caught them red-handed and ordered them out. However, Elmer and Sharon soon made up.

Sharon's life came to an abrupt end on the opening night of the grand tabernacle. The structure caught fire and she refused to leave. Others escaped, including Elmer, who did not heed Sharon's call to stay and try their faith.

He tried and failed as an independent evangelist. Then he joined a woman practicing 'New Thought' whose staff included a Hindu Swami. Interestingly, Elmer could play games more easily with 'New Thought' than with regular Protestantism because he was not afraid of the former. Monetary conflicts with his boss led him to try his own prosperity classes but they did not prosper.

Finally Elmer impressed a Methodist Bishop and became a minister of the Methodist church. He got a church and he met Cleo whom he married later. He was moving upward again. During his lean days Elmer borrowed some money from good old Frank Shallard. Frank had his doubts about the dogma of the church but he stuck with his ministry for family and financial reasons. He did not want to hurt his father, who was a minister, and Frank had to take care of his wife and children. Frank found consolation in a fellow Methodist preacher, Mr. Pengilly.

Mr. Pengilly had been a genuine shepherd to his flock for forty years; he was a true mystic, well versed in the Bible and in the Early Christian Fathers. His loving nature and his sense of humor were remarkable. He had loved his wife so dearly that after she died less than a year after their marriage, he did not look for any romantic involvement. Mr. Pengilly enjoyed nature. He could gently smile over the cranks among his flock. The differences between denominations were not important to him; what mattered was to work together for the betterment of all. Regarding the intelligent workmen who did not attend the church, Mr. Pengilly consoled Frank with a good-natured laugh. He even liked the village atheist and invited the atheist to his home. Although both were Methodist preachers, Mr. Pengilly's character was in sharp constrast to that of Elmer Gantry. The former showed features of mature spirituality— love, open-mindedness, knowledge, courage, prudence, and mature psychological defenses.

Elmer enjoyed his new found power and prestige. The ministerial role gave him outlets to satisfy his histrionic instincts. For a short time he even got interested in literature—Dickens, Longfellow, and Robert Burns. While these interests were mellowing him slightly, his Bishop urged him to read philosophy. The philosophy went over his head and brought his literary interests to a halt.

A clever salesman, he was good at raising money for the church. He kept up manly activities like going fishing and owning a dog, which gave him credibility among the men of the community. He kicked the dog when he was out in the country but poured attention on it when he was in town.

Elmer advertised his services with eye-catching phrases. He used every scare tactic to frighten his audience into following his preachings. He even induced his wife to promote his ambitious career by flattering her; he neglected or criticized her otherwise. He also dressed prim and proper.

He was a domineering husband. As he busied himself with building his holy empire, he paid little attention to his wife. Not only that, he embarrassed the innocent and shy Cleo. He had two children, a boy and a girl. Just one month after the little girl was born, Elmer wanted to make love to his wife but she was not ready. That infuriated Elmer so much that he slept in a separate bedroom from then on. His wife could not please him enough. His children were afraid of him even when he play-acted the role of a kind father one evening.

He found comfort in willing women parishioners or other women on his business trips. These escapades did not satisfy him; and besides it made him feel uneasy. The more intense his own inner conflicts were, the more furiously he condemned the same sins in his preaching. He raged against dancing, drinking, and movie going; and he condemned people who ran such businesses. These speeches made him popular; he attracted large crowds, and these results reinforced his behavior. While continuing his holy ascent, he came across his old flame Lulu, who had been married to Floyd for many years. They carried on a secret romance, often at the church.

As his power and popularity grew, so did his ambitious fight against immorality. He formed a committee on Public Morals and tried to enroll ministers of other denominations. He calculated they could join hands against sin,   although they detested one another. They enjoyed detailed discussions about manifestations of various sins. However no other minister favored Elmer's plans for witch hunts. The lack of support did not deter Elmer from going ahead single-handedly.

Elmer's ambition was never satisfied. He thought about becoming an Episcopalian to have more class; he dreamed of becoming a Bishop. He wished that his wife would die so that he could marry a more prominent woman.

He was a bigot but not a fool. He knew it would be foolish to support the Ku Klux Klan because of how the nice rich urban population would react. He personally believed in the principles of KKK but he was diplomatic in his public stance. He defended the freedom of every body to organize (including the KKK) and pleased both the KKK and its opponents.

One evening Elmer boasted to Mr. Pengilly about his achievements in the war against immoralists. It took the wisdom—and the impertinence—of a saintly Mr. Pengilly to ask Elmer the most pertinent question as to why he did not believe in God. Thickheaded Elmer did not understand the meaning of the question.

Elmer's evil reached its peak in the way he destroyed his old friend Frank. Through an old friend of Frank, Elmer learned about Frank's frustrations with the church and its hypocritical ministers. Elmer knew that a millionaire, Mr. Styles, was a member of Frank's church. With the cunning help of an attorney, Elmer set out to destroy Frank and catch the millionaire fish. Elmer contacted Mr. Styles and stirred up the congregation against Frank. Frank finally resigned.

Some covservative clergymen had noticed a decline in income and influence and formed well-funded organizations to scare legislators into passing laws forbidding teaching anything in schools that the evangelists did not approve. They were threatened by authentic learning in biology, history, astronomy, and psychology. A few groups of scholars opposed such censorhip. Frank gave a speech to one of these groups. He was kidnapped and beaten up for it. His eyes were damaged so severely that he could not read again, an activity that he had cherished dearly.

Continuing his ascent, Elmer became one of the first radio preachers in the country. That brought him more fame and huge collections. He traveled to Europe once but found the foreigners had no 'git up and git'. His career climaxed with offers from a famous Methodist church in New York to become its pastor, and from the National Association for the Purification of Art and the Press to become its secretary. He accepted both offers.

Although he got into trouble because of his amorous relationship with his secretary, his attorney friend outwitted her and saved the situation. The book ends with Elmer's prayer (temporarily distracted by his eyes falling on a beautiful choir girl) to make the United States "a moral nation."

The whole story of Elmer Gantry's religiosity is shot through with unhealthy elements. Fear was its most prominent aspect during his early life. Later on, he was more motivated by pride and greed as well as hate of opponents. He used fear to convert other people into good behavior. One instance illustrates how fear leads to excessive control. The Dean of Terwillinger College cautioned a faculty friend about approving soft drinks because people might slip from giner ale to ale. While Elmer had excessive fear in one way, he lacked healthy moral anxiety about his evil intentions and wrongdoings.

He certainly did not love his enemies; he did not evn love his family or friends. Other people were just tools for his power and pleasure. He lacked empathic understanding of others but he knew how to manipulate them. Compassion had no place in his personal life or his religious preaching. On the other hand, he was a strong hater. With that hate he destroyed people whose views and ways were different from his own.

Ignorance was at the root of his problems. The narrow world view from his childhood was not significantly changed by his college education. His seminary education left a lot to be desired in terms of enlightening his mind. Instead, it sanctified his narrow outlook. Sacking of the scholarly Dr. Zechlin from the seminary, and the evangelists trying to control school education, are examples of how narrow views are perpetuated. The search for truth, and for mystical experience, had little place in the fanatical world of Hallelujah yells, money making, religious empire-building, and destroying enemies. Neither transformation of oneself into authentic selfhood nor attempts at transforming evildoers were given a chance.

Identity of Elmer was clearly focused on his gender, race, nationality, and his version of Christianity. In sharp contrast was the universal identity of Mr. Pengilly. While Elmer was a fanatic and Mr. Pengilly a mystic, Frank Shallard was somewhere in between. Frank did not have the courage, wisdom, and healthy self-love to become authentic and integrated. He wasted away those potentials, remaining spiritually and emotionally half-baked; but he did not degenerate into a fanatic to gain security or admiration from fanatic followers.

With Faith and Fury   is a captivating novel with interesting characters and an open discussion of philosophical issues on religion, particularly Christianity. The power of human sexuality is a persistent theme entering into many of the intrapsychic as well as interpersonal connections and conflicts in the story. For a fanatic Freudian, the entire book can be seen as a matter of repressed sexuality. From a broad perspective, there is a lot more that the book teaches as it also delights the reader with its wit and wisdom. However, a mystic like Mr. Pengilly or a spiritually half-baked Frank Shallard as in *Elmer Gantry* are absent. Prominently present, though, is an agnostic young professor of philosophy, Adrian Dewulf, who may be the mouthpiece of the author himself.

Manly John Plumwell grew up in the small town of Nickel Plate. His grandparents raised him after his parents died in a plane crash. He was a loner. Manly was considered a good boy by all and sundry. Although he had experimented with cigar butts at the early age of about two and a half, he had given up any such vices as he grew a few years older.

As a teenager Manly found renewed temptations to smoke. More than that he had entirely new temptations of the flesh—impure thoughts, the craving to drink, and the urge to masturbate. He was too shy to enter into any biological experiments with girls, too shy even to take some girls on a ride to the county fair. When he was eighteen and about to be a senior in high school, he secretly watched a burlesque show at the county fair. Luckily, or perhaps unluckily, a show girl fell down from the platform and ended up in his lap. That was one of the high marks of his youth—too low a mark for most youth these days.

That night when he was sleeping blissfully after a wet dream about the dancing girl, Manly was awakened by screams from his grandmother. He tried to get the sole county doctor to come to her rescue, but the old lady's soul departed before the doctor arrived. The tender conscience of Manly coupled with his magical, irrational thinking made him feel that his sinfulness caused her death.

Manly was interested in religious matters even as a child. The Plumwells belonged to the denomination Disciples of Christ. They believed in adult baptism but Manly had pushed his grandmother to get him baptized years before he became an adult. He believed that baptism was a ticket to heaven.

Manly was slowly recovering from the grief and guilt over his grandmother's death. He had graduated from high school. His future was uncertain. At such a time of stress, two young men—priests of the Holy Nation Association—approached him to join their ranks. They impressed Manly with their talks about the wicked world racing towards disaster, Commander Jesus Christ, the spirit-filled lives of the members of the Holy Nation, and the like. Manly agreed to accompany them to meet the handmaiden of the Lord, Miss Alice McAlister, who founded this sect. He was promptly accepted into the group.

Ms McAlister became the founder of a new Christian denomination on the basis of some new interpretations of the Bible. A lonely child with religious inclinations, one night during her sleepwalk she stumbled upon her parents making love. An intense reaction followed, beginning with extreme withdrawal and ending with her emergence preaching a new version of Christianity. She vehemently repressed sexuality in herself and her followers. Using all the techniques of her profession, she organized a successful church with many branches and with headquarters at Big Bend. According to the novelist, they started with credulity, passed through belief in the plausible, and ended up with a faith that could transform fiction into fact and vice versa.

They claimed the literal truth of their interpretation of the Bible; they also claimed all other interpretations and all other scriptures in the world as the work of the devil. They had no use for philosophy, psychology, and such other perversions of degenerate minds. In their prayers and daily lives, they emphasized the fear of the Lord. The more they emptied themselves of personal worth, the more they filled themselves with divine vanity. The more they readied themselves to be sacrificial lambs for the glory of their faith, the more grandiose they became.

After his training at Big Bend and a failed mission as minister at Calico corners, Manly was assigned to minister to his own folks in Nickel Plate. He was great at conducting funerals. Manly conducted the wedding ceremonies well enough, but the after-effects of it were disastrous; he was sexually stimulated without satisfactory outlets.

Because of the scarcity of hardcore sins in Nickel Plate to keep him busy and to extend the influence of the Holy Nation further afield, Manly extended his evangelistic action to nearby Dewmaker. The focus of his attention was the dance hall of Dewmaker, which bred sensuality. He could not stop the people from enjoying dancing. On the contrary, he became so entranced by a nineteen-year-old beauty that he made sexual advances towards her (in vain). While his sensuality was getting out of control, as evidenced in his attempt to peep at young women as they changed clothes after baptism, Manly was encouraged by the leaders of the Holy Nation to join Algonquin State University for higher education and to spread their influence to the campus. Manly went along: he found fertile soil for sowing the seeds of the Holy Nation in the immature minds of many students.

Adrian Dewulf, a young professor of philosophy, and a former minister, was the biggest challenger to Manly. He had left the ministry because he could not honestly believe what he was supposed to believe and preach to others. Confronting the fraudulent followers of religion became a personal passion for him. Adrian's passionate dislike for religion and Manly's passionate belief in the Holy Nation clashed on several occasions. One of Adrian's admirers was a beautiful student, Clare Sumner, who attended Manly's church.

Manly, the local shepherd of the Holy Nation, had special interest in this particular sheep. He was sexually attracted to her but he was not *manly* enough to deal openly with it. He enjoyed seeing her in the congregation or in any situation. A budding love relationship between Clare and a Catholic boy was known to Manly, and he had plans to break it up. Clare was growing intellectually. She had many interesting discussions with Adrian. Gradually Adrian lowered his defenses and let Clare get close to him. Finally they became lovers. Manly knew from direct observation and from reports of a student who worked as a secret agent that his ultimate foe and the apple of his eye had become intimate.

In the meantime, Manly had attempted to convert Adrian by first trying to humiliate him. The attempt only boomeranged. Confrontations with Adrian left Manly doubtful of some of his own beliefs. He became obsessed with some of Adrian's attacks on Christendom. Finally the combination of jealousy and the need to punish an evil sinner pushed Manly over the edge to commit the cold-blooded murder of Adrian. The fear and hate generated by Adrian shaking up his belief system, as well as the sense of impotence in his twin failure to win Clare sexually or spiritually, must have been important factors in Manly's ultimately cowardly act.

As Manly's hideous crime was discovered, the Holy Nation dropped him like a hot potato, leaving him to fend for himself. He was sentenced to life imprisonment. Three and a half years later he was transferred to a state hospital for the criminally insane, where he belonged more properly.

The dynamics of fear, neurotic guilt, narrow foci of identity, and hate are certainly noticeable in the novel. However, the problems of ignorance and the evil consequence of repressed sexuality are far more clearly depicted. Manly's problems in the areas of knowledge and will are beautifully summarized: "While still very young, he murdered his own mind so as to enjoy the salvation of certitude. He aspired to serve a sovereign who would permit him to superimpose his own powerful will upon others while appearing to be a mere servant."[1]

Life, it is said, is stranger than fiction. The facts about Jim Jones and the phenomenon of cults in the next chapter may prove to be so in comparison to the two works of fiction we dealt with here.

14 . JIM JONES AND CULT PHENOMENA

"I don't claim to be god, but millions of people say I am." — Father Divine

The news of the mass suicide-homicide of nine hundred and thirteen people (including Jones) in Jonestown, Guyana on November 18, 1978, shocked the whole world. It is one of the most bizarre episodes in the history of the human race, and a stark example of unhealthy religiosity.

Reverend James Warren Jones and his followers who constituted the People's Temple cult decided to act out on that fateful day the 'white night' they had rehearsed for some time. It is hardly surprising that they carried out the grotesque ritual under the circumstances, because they were well prepared for it. Far more surprising is the kind of thinking and planning that had gone on actively among so many people. The power of fanatical faith is hard to believe. But then human beings have shown such propensities time and again. In fact, a Baptist minister said that the preparation for a nuclear war is the clearest example of the Jonestown phenomenon on a massive scale.

Just dubbing Jones as a devil who caught hundreds of innocent people in the net of his vices is simplistic and untrue. Equally false is the contention of some christian fundamentalists that it was not religion but Marxism that caused the problems of Jones. Moreover, to interpret all of Jim Jones' actions as evil because of the evil deeds of his last few years also misses the right perspective. In looking for the dark devil with two horns and a tail, we miss the real human evil which is often mixed with varying degrees of goodness. Attributing all the responsibility to the cult leader is to deny the role of the followers and the silent witnesses. The Jonestown tragedy has opened people's eyes to the danger of cultism. It ought to open people's minds to the wider issues involved.

James W. Jones was born on May 13, 1931, in Lynn, a small town in Indiana. He was the only child of James and Lynetta Jones. The older Jones suffered from respiratory problems because he was gassed in World War I. He drew a disability check from the government. Because of his illness, the father did not spend much time with the son.

Lynetta Jones had to work in a factory and at odd jobs to supplement the family income. Even then, they could barely make both ends meet. Before marrying, she had worked as an anthropologist in Africa for a while. She had given up her career to follow a dream she had. In that dream, she saw her mother telling her that Lynetta would give birth to a boy who would right the wrongs of the world. So she had great expectations for little Jim.

The little town of Lynn was interesting in at least two respects: its main industry was casket making, and it had a strong following of the Ku Klux Klan. In fact, the older Jones was a member of the KKK. The town had six churches.

Little Jones was lonely, an only child, with a sick father and a working mother. From his early years, he showed an inclination to religion. He enjoyed pretending to be a preacher. He went to different churches as his whims and fancies took him. One neighbor introduced him to the Nazarene faith.

Jim followed his mother's example of using curse words. He did not have many friends. Jim showed certain unusual interests as a youth, taking care of stray animals and conducting funeral services for dead pets. His preoccupation with suffering and death was obvious. He had a short temper. And he was bold and individualistic like his mother, who was reportedly the first woman in her town to smoke cigarettes openly.

He gave his first sermon in a black church at age fourteen. Although he did not participate in sports, he organized them at times. He did not care to be an ordinary participant in anything; he had to play a leading role. This urge indicates paranoid tendency to be in control so that he could be sure how matters would shape up.

In school he was only an average student but his I.Q. was 115 to 120. During his senior year in high school, he had to work. While other boys chased girls, Jim pursued religion. He changed schools after his sophomore year because he did not like the racist attitude in Lynn. He graduated from the school in Richmond, a larger town close by. His interest in becoming a minister grew stronger.

In 1949 he entered Indiana University. While working as an orderly in a local hospital, he met Merceline Baldwin, a nurse four years older than himself. They married the same year. There is speculation that she was a mother figure for him which, if true, is not surprising because his mother did not meet his affectional needs satisfactorily as a child.

In the following year, he and his wife moved to Indianapolis and he became pastor at a racially integrated local church. He had dropped out of Indiana University. He became an ordained minister many years later—in 1964—in a branch of the Disciples of Christ.

At a time and in a place where racism was strong, Jim Jones opposed it. Consequently, conservative members caused him problems; he had to change churches several times. The KKK also caused him problems. He faced these difficulties courageously and was all the more respected.

In 1956 he opened his own church, the People's Temple in Indianapolis. By then he had adopted seven children of black, white, and Asian descent. He also encouraged his congregation to be actively compassionate. He identified with the poor and the downtrodden and worked hard to help them. Coming from a background of bigotry, his strong desire for racial integration was really remarkable.

In 1961 the city of Indianapolis recognized his good works and made him the director of the city's Human Rights Commission. A largely decorative position, it nevertheless became a podium from which he could sell himself and his mission. Everything seemed to be going well. But he was looking for innovations and improvements in style and substance; so he visited the churches of famous preachers and observed their mode of action. That route took him gradually down hill to the ultimate disaster.

In order to understand the course of Jim Jones's life from around the early 1960's, one has to recognize the significance of the political position he was given by the city and the influence of a preacher called Father Divine in his life. The political position whetted his appetite for more fame and power as he also gained an understanding of how good works can bring rich rewards. The tactics of Father Divine became a model for Jones to follow.

Father Divine was an interesting phenomenon in the American religious scene. His Kingdom of Peace movement reportedly had a million followers by the late 1950's. His followers believed him to be the Messiah. The son of a black sharecropper, he grew up in Georgia. As a young man, he was active in a religious movement called "Live Forever, Die Forever" and for that he was found guilty by the state officials and given the choice of leaving the state or being committed to a state mental hospital. He chose the former. In 1915 he started preaching and doing social service in Harlem.

He was charged with disturbing the peace and brought before a judge in the 1920's. He told the judge that the latter would die and three days later the judge died of a heart attack. This incident convinced his followers of his divinity. The poor were given food and shelter in the 'Heavens' he set up gradually in various parts of the country. Initially he raised money by collecting a part of the income of the people for whom he found employment. Later, he asked new members to turn over their savings to him. At the time of his death, the Kingdom of Peace was estimated to be worth ten million dollars.

Father Divine's success and grandiosity left a strong impression on the impressionable Jones. Many of Divine's techniques were adopted by Jones—healing of the sick was one. Divine had an inner circle of loyalists, an interrogation committee to safeguard his power from the potential and actual troublemakers among his followers. While Divine preached purity of body and mind, he was accused of seducing members of his flock. He apparently rationalized his actions as part of his religious duty to bring out and eliminate the desires of the people involved.

Reverend Jones started a healing ministry. He faked miracles with the conniving assistance of a few loyalists. Rotting chicken livers were used as cancerous growths he was bringing out from the victims of cancer. Faith healing is indeed one of the surest ways to become a rich and famous minister, as so many have proven. Jones set up an interrogation committee which became more and more punitive in the years to come. Somewhere down the road Jones also started sexual exploitation and control of his followers.

Though his religious enterprise was booming, criticism erupted over his faith healing. With his finances growing fast, Jones set up two corporations—one a non-profit corporation and the other a family enterprise. However, he was not successful with these ventures and had to give them up. Moreover, the ventures caused conflicts with governmental authorities over his failure to file annual reports etc. The atmosphere of Indianapolis was becoming less supportive of Jones' enterprises. At the same time he began to fear a nuclear war; he had visions of a nuclear holocaust. He had read a magazine article that listed the ten safest places to live in case of a nuclear war; Ukiah, California was one of them. It is also quite likely that Jones sensed a better opportunity for his sect in California. With all these factors in favor of a move to Ukiah, Jones and company took that very step in November 1965.

At Ukiah, Jones and his followers did an excellent public relations job. They won friends and influenced people by their work. Jones got on the good side of the media by awarding grants; he impressed the police and public officials by charitable works and won the hearts of the public by good deeds. His devout followers were easily available for political rallies, making him a political force to be reckoned with. The People's Temple operated a boys home, three convalescent centers, a pet shelter, and several foster homes. Mrs. Jones became the state nursing home inspector.

By then, Jones had something to offer almost everyone. He had shelters for the homeless, food for the starving, meaning for the meaningless, sense of belonging for the rootless, political support for the politicians, healing for the sick, and miracles for the gullible. He was the "Father" to his followers; he did not claim to be God.

His fame and fortune continued to grow in the favorable soil of California. So did his psychopathology under the influence of more power and prestige. He became all the more dictatorial, philandering, sadistic, and suspicious of others. Several armed security guards were working to protect him. When questioned about this, Jones claimed that this was the decision of his church leaders in spite of his own preference to the contrary. In Indiana, when he was asked about submitting the cancer specimen he was taking out from patient's bodies, he had dodged the issue with the same excuse that his church leaders did not want more publicity and he reluctantly went along with them.

In a few years Ukiah was too small for Jones's operations. So he moved to San Francisco in 1972. He continued his public relations ploys so successfully that in 1976 he was made Chairman of the Housing Authority. In the meantime, Jones was still searching for the paradise on Earth where he could settle down for good. He chose a place near Georgetown, Guyana. The low cost of living, the use of English as the official language, a socialist government, people who seemed ripe for his ministry, and expectation of protection from nuclear or racial holocaust were special attractions of Guyana for Jones. Beginning in 1974, the People's Temple gradually moved to Jonestown, Guyana. Most of the People's Temple members and Jones himself were in Jonestown by the end of 1977.

After hearing about the beatings, sexual abuses, and suicide drills of the Jonestown cult for over a year, Congressman Leo Ryan, a Democrat from California, decided to investigate the matter. He arrived for that purpose in Guyana in November 1978. On November 18, 1978, as he ws returning to the United States with some members of the People's Temple who wanted to leave the cult, Jones' lieutenants attacked and killed Congressman Ryan and several others. That same day Jonestown members enacted the gruesome 'white night'—the suicide ritual.

Babies were given cyanide first and they died fast. Then older children were lined up and given cups of kool-aid mixed with cyanide. Parents of the children and older people followed suit. Armed guards made sure the process went smoothly and nobody escaped. The guards and Jones must have been among the last to go. In keeping with his special stature, he died of a bullet rather than the cyanide drink. It is uncertain whether he died by suicide or homicide. While all this was going on, his tape-recorded message was encouraging the people to follow the ritual, even promising to meet in another place.

Thus ended one of the strangest religious cults. After the demise of the cult, revelations about what went on within the group became public, secrets unraveling from the few members who survived because they were away that day or from people who had left the group previously. That information, coupled with the history of the man, gives us fair insight into the dynamics of Jones and his followers. Jim Jones showed the characteristics of a religious fanatic. We will take up these one by one.

He was very vain—narcissistic. Jones paid special attention to his appearance—he dyed his hair, wore nice clothes, and boasted about his attractiveness. He had a bodyguard to carry a suitcase of make-up materials. Power and control over members of his cult was something he relished. For him, sexuality became a proof of his prowess and power over others. His secretary arranged for him to have sexual relations with whomever among his flock he chose, much like a king used his harem in the royal days. He had homosexual relations too. When a young woman was having her period, Jones forced a middle-aged man to have oral sex with her. Jones showed what is called "polymorphous perverse sexuality" in psychiatric jargon. He demanded special treatment in his diet and special protection by his guards. Adoration from followers was essential for him; he used every opportunity to show off.

Besides being proud, he was greedy. He was never satisfied with what he had—he wanted to expand more and more. He even dreamed about becoming a big political leader. While he greedily took in everything the cult members had, he was reluctant to give them more than the bare necessities of life. The followers slavishly accepted his greed.

Fear was very much a central dynamic of Jones. He always feared other people and government agencies. His elaborate secrecies and personal guards bore witness to that fear. Jones moved from place to place as much out of paranoia (including fear of racial and nuclear holocausts) as to expand his operations. His preoccupation with death was obvious even as a child conducting funeral services for dead animals. The suicide drills he practiced in the commune showed the ultimate height of his fears. The murder of the Congressman and the final massacre of his followers topped it off. Narcissism as well as aggression and control are manifestations of unhealthy ways of handling fear of death, as we noted earlier. So also can be excessive sexual indulgence. (As we saw in Chapter 5)

While Jones suffered from excessive fear, he did not have the prudence that goes with a good conscience. He could lie, cheat, break any commandment of his Christian faith, and completely disregard the golden rule without a prick of conscience. His fear was about other people finding out, of being exposed.

He showed courage in promoting racial integration in a community that was racist. Apart from this, he did not show courage in any important aspects of life—certainly no courage to be open to the criticism of others or to search for truth and wisdom or to love genuinely.

He remained largely ignorant, never even seeking to acquire a proper seminary education. Little of his time was devoted to genuine learning after he dropped out of the University. With ignorance and a closed mind, he fed on his own illusions. Prominent among his illusions were those dreams of establishing an ideal society in a paradise on earth using his peculiar techniques.

His fundamentalist mindset was a root cause of such problems. Shiv Naipaul observed in *Journey to Nowhere:* "The People's Temple was laid out on the latitudinal and longitudinal grid of the fundamentalist imagination; an imagination obsessed with sin and images of apocalyptic destruction, authoritarian in its innermost impulses, instinctively thinking in terms of the saved and the damned, seeking not to enlighten but to terrorize into obedience."[1]

He hated anybody and everybody who stood in his way to power and glory. He hated government agencies, a critical media, neighbors who complained, and followers who questioned him. His sadism was an expression of his hate.

The sadist enjoys forcing emotional and physical pain on others. It gives the sadist an additional sense of power and control. It is the opposite of love; when we love, we try to give enjoyment and pleasure to the ones we love. Jones enjoyed humiliating and beating the members of his cult in public. Some sadists—and Jones was one—particularly enjoy preying on the weak ones. He enjoyed the sights of children being cruelly punished, even beaten with cattle prods. His destructiveness was of course most clearly and definitely demonstrated in the mass suicide-homicide.

His followers manifested blind obedience, excessive fear, lack of self-respect, masochism, lack of genuine love for others, and self-destructiveness. Otherwise they would not have stayed with him through all the madness that was going on. When any of the members disagreed with Jones, other members took up Jones's side, thereby reinforcing conformism in the group. The members shared in Jones's evil doings actively and passively. *They committed spiritual suicide long before they killed themselves physically.*

It behooves us here to understand the cult phenomena in general. There is currently a considerable body of literature in the mental health field to help us in that process. For our purpose I will summarize some of the most pertinent views about cults. I will base it largely on several writings of psychiatrist Saul V. Levine and the book *Cults in America* by anthropoligist Willa Appel.

In an article in *Canadian Journal of Psychiatry* (December 1981) Dr. Levine made several important points based on considerable research, literature review, and clinical work. Some of his conclusions are contrary to popular notions. For example he found that, compared to other dedicated and demanding movements, cults do not attract the more clinically disturbed population nor affect the members more adversely. Cults were found to meet certain important needs such as believing and belonging and to show certain beneficial effects:

> Reduction in anxiety and depression in people who experienced it prior to joining the cult.

> At times provide a helpful milieu for members with emotional or behavioral problems.

> Alleviate alienation, poor self-esteem, and feelings of demoralization.

Even individuals who are significantly emotionally disturbed benefit from the acceptance of a group with clearcut structure, obvious expectations, and emotional support. In trying to help the severely disturbed individuals, some cults cooperate with psychiatric services whereas others do not.

Only about one out of eight people who visit a cult joins it. After a member leaves the cult, symptoms often develop. A variety of negative feelings (guilt, depression, anxiety, confusion, etc.) may be experienced. Moreover, the original cause that led to joining the cult may reappear with renewed strength.

Cults cause or contribute to disturbing patterns of thought and behavior. These include unquestioning reverence for the leader and his/her teachings, intolerance of other points of view, and rejection of past relationships (family, friends, etc.). There is a strong tendency toward anti-intellectualism, leading to the blocking of psychological and social development. Lack of adaptive flexibility and insensitivity to others' needs are also unwelcome changes.

Levine's book *Radical Departures* is subtitled *Desperate Detours to Growing Up,* indicating an empathetic view of cults. The author argues persuasively that the radical departure—leaving one's home and community to join a cult—is a detour in the process of growing up. The detour is a result of the blockage of normal paths to growing up—a blockage caused by society's failure to meet youth's need for believing and belonging.

More than ninety percent of those who join the cults return to their families within two years. Moreover, those who return home pick up the threads of their lives and move on to become well-adjusted citizens. Those who voluntarily leave the cults keep some of the new-found values that can be well integrated into their lives such as faith and altruism.

Deprogramming does not work most of the time and when it does the results are worse. Members of cults who are deprogrammed become hostile towards their former cults. These individuals not only fail to integrate any of the useful values of their former cult, they continue to manifest fanatical tendencies. Levine is not recommending cultism. He acknowledges the pain and sufferings the families of cult members go through as well as the loss of valuable time and resources to the members and to society at large. Moreover, a strong potential exists for a cult leader with significant psychopathology to lead the followers into various forms of destructiveness as in the Jonestown case. In fact, Levine points out better alternatives for youths, their families, and for society: programs like the Mormon Church's youth service, Canada's Katimavik program, and the Peace Corps of the United States.

At least one group of people does not benefit from joining, classified as runaways. Usually younger in age, the runaways join cults to escape from destructive homes. These individuals are often emotionally troubled; their psychological defenses are not strong. Although they show temporary improvements, they do not seem to make healthy and lasting changes by joining cults. Levine does not explain what happens to those who do not drop out of the cults.

In the book *Psychodynamic Perspectives on Religion, Sect and Cult*, Levine has contributed a chapter entitled *Alienated Jewish Youth and Religious Seminaries: An Alternative to Cults?*. The chapter is based on extensive interviews of one hundred and ten young Jewish men from the United States, Canada, and other countries who had left their families and lifestyles and entered Orthodox Jewish seminaries in Israel. Eighty to ninety percent of them were from upper middle class and non-orthodox backgrounds. Jewish fundamentalism was a new discovery for them. They were not drop-outs of society but skilled intelligent young men. In spite of the fact that these men were joining Jewish seminaries, their families were unhappy. The achievement-oriented parents viewed their sons' choices as undesirable. Levine found that the young men's need for believing and belonging was met by their lives in the seminaries.

Willa Appel emphasizes the problematic aspects of the cults. She points out that cults, now more than ever before, are greater in number and also in wealth and power. Cults set themselves apart in showing varying degrees of hostility towards the outside world. Cults are often led by charismatic and authoritarian figures. Members of a cult fervently follow a certain ideology; doubts and questions about the ideology are repressed or suppressed. Appel's analysis of the stages of conversion and the psychological techniques used are both convincing and important for our purposes.

The first of the three stages of conversion consists of isolation of the individual from his or her past relationships, occupation, etc. Physical and emotional distancing from family and friends serves this purpose. In the second phase, the individual is pushed to surrender his or her past life using guilt and humiliation. For example guilt and humiliation about one's life before entering the cult and all real and imaginary evils of one's society are used to impress upon the newcomer the need to surrender the past. In the next stage, the joiner is given a new identity along with a new philosophy of life. These stages are part and parcel of any conversion, be it evangelical born-again experience, joining a cult, or communist thought-reform practiced in China.

Old and new techniques are used by cults in attracting and maintainig converts. The time-honored religious practices that produce trance-like stages, ecstacy by chanting, speaking in tongues, dancing, and the like are well utilized. The confrontational therapeutic approaches of encounter groups is another technique used by cults. And in a world of marketing, cults are adept at using high-powered sales tactics. These techniques are used by religious revivalists also.

Appel observes that conversion tactics of the cults produce a dissociative stage in the newcomer, making it easy for the ideology of the cult to be accepted by the potential convert. As a hypnotherapist, I would say this is a clever utilization of hypnotic techniques in a non-therapeutic way.

Cults exploit individuals and pose a danger to society. Members of many cults are ready and willing to go to any extremes to protect their power and position. Like religious revivals, cults may challenge the established order of religion and society and lead to reforms and renewals for the better. But there are far better ways of reform than through cults.

In an overview of studies on charismatic religious sects (*American Journal of Psychiatry,* December, 1982) Marc Galanter notes that those who join sects show limited social ties and psychological distress before joining a sect. Remission in substance abuse is one beneficial effect in joining sects that denounce drug use. Group cohesion and control of boundary is achieved through maintaining the distinctive characteristics of the sect, from ideology to dress and customs. Also members are closely monitored. Members reinforce each other's beliefs and customs.

The danger of cults was demonstrated in 1985 when some aides of Bhagvan Rajneesh committed crimes such as wiretapping, poisoning, salmonella poisoning, and setting fire to Wasco County Planning Office. There was talk of potential for a blood bath. Fortunately the Rajneesh sect in Oregon was dismantled without further escalations, thanks to timely governmental action.

If we hark back to the existential concerns human beings are faced with (as we saw in Chapter V), it is easy to recognize that cults do meet the existential needs, although in unhealthy ways. The issues of isolation, freedom, and responsibility are met by fusion with the group. The fears of death and meaninglessness are alleviated by deep involvement in group activities and adherence to the belief system of the cult. However, authenticity and other healthy ways of dealing with existential dilemmas are basically absent or weak.

The experiences of the self-help group Fundamentalists Anonymous (F.A.) is also worth considering here. In its one year of existence, over 17,000 ex-fundamentalists have sought help from F.A. According to Richard Yao, founder of F. A., the root problems of fundamentalism is "the fundamentalist mindset"—one of authoritarianism, intolerance and compulsion to control, and an either/or mentality. Mr. Yao, a New York attorney, is a former christian fundamentalist who abjured fundamentalism during his studies at Yale Divinity School.

F.A. helps those who wish to leave fundamentalism and experience problems in doing so. The common problems of ex-fundamentalists are those of *depression* (self blame, low self-esteem, loneliness), *fear* (fear of Divine retribution, fear of harassment from fundamentalists, chronic distrust of people), bitterness over wasted time, lapses into former mindset, inability to talk about their traumatic experience with fundamentalism, and sexual dysfunctions. According to F.A., fundamentalist groups and religious cults are similar except the former have more power and clout. Reportedly, it takes at least three years on the average really to leave fundamentalism. (My personal view of fundamentalism is expressed in Chapter 4 .) The adverse effects reported by those who leave religious cults or fundamentalism are similar to the after-effects of traumatic experiences such as rape and assault. These after-effects show the traumatic nature of cultism.

While religious cults can show some beneficial effects, they are also pregnant with potential dangers. While such groups may often profess the virtues of love, courage, prudence, and wisdom, their practices often show exactly the opposite dynamics. At the weak points in their lives, people are more vulnerable to becoming victims of such unhealthy religiosity. Young people going through a difficult stage in life are, therefore, easy prey to cult leaders like Jones. In the last decade and a half of his life, Jim Jones personified religious fanaticism.

15. FROM DARKNESS TO LIGHT

Case of Joanne. Joanne was referred to me by her internist for treatment of depression, anxiety, and severe tension headaches. She was in her early fifties. Her symptoms were a result of several major stresses in her life: one of her teenage daughters indulged in sexual promiscuity; her job had become more stressful because of new computerized systems; her father had become more irritating and belittling. She had a strong family history of depression and therefore a genetic component also to her problem.

She was a perfectionist, rigid and set in her ways, with an extreme sense of right and wrong and a very strict conscience. Because she perceived failure in many areas of her life, she was burdened with enormous neurotic guilt. Being an intelligent person with much curiosity, she had doubts about her rigid christian beliefs; but she never dared to explore the questions because of fear of God's wrath.

However, she was open to the possibility of better spirituality because she was dissatisfied with her attempt to fit in the mold of the "true Christians", according to what she learned as she was growing up.

She had to be hospitalized because of the severity of her condition. Along with medications for depression and anxiety, regular psychotherapy and group threrapy, I recommended that she read *The Road Less Traveled* by Scott Peck and *Reconciliations* by Theodore Rubin. She enjoyed both but found the former book much more useful. She reread, underlined, and sidemarked several parts of the first book and asked my help to apply those ideas to her life. This was a great opening for her spiritual growth.

After this, I slowly presented to her, briefly, my ideas about the healthy and unhealthy aspects of religion. That clarified a lot of her confusion. Interestingly, during that time she had a wonderful dream: from a distance she was seeing God seated on his throne and he was glorious; then, she got nearer and took a close look at him and realized he had two horns and a tail; and he was holding a pitchfork in his hands. As we explored this dream, she quickly recognized how her concept of God was of a demonic figure full of wrath and ready to send millions of people to eternal damnation for petty human frailties. Fear was the most predominant aspect of her religion followed by a narrow outlook and pride in her denomination. As we worked on her fears, it became clear that she had considerable problems in loving because of her self-hate. A major cause of the self-hate was her sense of unworthiness and guilt based on her mistaken

188

religious ideas. She took responsibility for the real and imagined wrongs of her family members as well as her own. In situations in which other people would be angry, she would become hateful of herself and have severe headaches. As she learned about these problems and worked on them, she became more loving.

Joanne improved sufficiently in three weeks to be sent home and followed up regularly on an outpatient basis. During the hospitalizations she had laid a good foundation for spiritual growth. She also had dreams about demolishing old structures and building on a new foundation. After a while, she was able to go back to work. She has continued follow-up treatments with medication and psychotherapy. And she has pursued her spiritual quest with further reading, group studies, spiritual workshops, and the like. She has become far more understanding, loving, courageous, and prudent. She is quite open-minded now and has a universal identity. This spiritual growth, she says, is the most cherished experience (series of experiences) of her life. She did not just get over her symptoms; she was reborn in the best sense of the word. She once said, "I really started living only when I began therapy."

Spouse of a Religious Fundamentalist. Let us call her Helen. She was in her thirties when she was referred to me by another physician who was treating her for various physical complaints. She was depressed and anxious. This attractive, young, white female had an unhappy childhood because of the economic hardship of the family and because of the marital conflicts of her parents. She had developed a spirit of autonomy and optimism on the surface but had strong dependency needs and deep insecurities.

Problems with her husband were the major psychological conflict for Helen at the time she consulted me. Her husband had, over the previous few years, gotten deeply involved with a Christian Church with very dogmatic beliefs, rigid attitudes, and puritanical practices. Helen had artistic interest and enjoyed singing, reading poetry and novels, and dancing. Her husband found these objectionable and put up blocks as much as he could. The obvious suffering of his wife and children, even Helen's overt emotional problems, did not make her husband take a critical look at his actions. Instead, he rationalized his actions all the more, quoting scripture profusely. This increased Helen's fury because she saw his attitude as hypocrisy.

Helen's husband was brought up by his father (who was a minister) in strict religious belief and practice, and had followed this after a period of rebellion in his youth. In fact he seemed to overcompensate for the rebellion of his youth by becoming even more extreme in his fundamentalism than his father had been. Helen was religious in the better sense of the word. Hers was more of a healthy spirituality but the fanaticism of her husband started to shake her religious faith itself. Many a time she was at the point of "shoving the whole thing and taking off somewhere."

In helping Helen, I explained my understanding of healthy spirituality and sick religiosity. My explanation made a lot of difference in Helen's understanding of her husband's and her own religious beliefs and of the way she could make things better for herself and her family. While mentally preparing to face divorce if her husband's fanatical tendencies persisted as an intolerable problem, Helen became more understanding and compassionate. While being assertive about some of her wishes, she showed genuine love and care toward her husband. She also began to love herself more as she realized what healthy spirituality is, and progressed further in her healthy tendencies. Her symptoms of depression and anxiety had cleared by then, but she continued to see me to help her with further emotional and spiritual growth. Gradually her husband became more secure and more open. He benefited significantly from Helen's healthy spirituality and became less fanatical.

As she was making progress, but before her condition became stable, Helen had a "peak experience." She was under considerable stress at that time because of children's sickness, her husband's job changes, and financial problems as well as some problems going on with her parents. One day she felt hopeless and thought of taking an overdose of medication. As she was seriously considering that action, thoughts like "Is there a God?", "Why is this happening to me?", "If things are going to be like this it is better for me to go to sleep" went through her mind. Then she felt a sudden jolt and sensed somebody in the room. She felt like a little child and felt God embracing her. All this happened in a flash. Everything she learned in her sessions with me and from her hospital stays and her readings came together, and she experienced a wholeness and deep sense of meaning in her life. Her suicidal ideations cleared and her depression went away.

Compulsive Salesman Burdened With Guilt. This patient, a salesman in his late forties, was depressed off-and-on for many years. In fact, he had been tried on different antidepressant medications and on Lithium. He was diagnosed as having manic depressive illness—depressed type. His was an obsessive compulsive personality—rigid, hard-driving, perfectionist, unable to relax and obsessed about past mistakes and future concerns. His parents were fanatic Christians who were constantly warning of God's wrath. As a child, he was taught how God would punish him for an infraction of the Ten Commandments, especially any sexual indiscretion. Masturbation was going to bring severe punishment in terms of severe physical and/or mental suffering.

During his teenage years, he suffered from compulsive masturbation. The more he was afraid of it, the worse it got. Then he married and things got better for a while but he and his wife gradually started having problems. His wife was more insecure and more rigid than himself. They both needed support, but rather than helping each other they grew apart. He also had problems at his work because of paying too much attention to minor details and delaying more important work. He was unhappy with his life. While working away from home, he had one sexual encounter with a woman, and that left him with intense guilt. The old guilt about masturbation also surfaced and with it came fear of divine retribution. Confessions, contritions, prayers, and penance all left him still quite dissatisfied with himself. He was preoccupied with guilt and fear of eternal damnation. However, he gradually got better with treatment and was able to work.

He had recurrent episodes of depression, beginning around the anniversary of his affair, but not every year. This went on for over six years. At this time his doctors were considering electric shock therapy, so he came to me for a second opinion. When he started seeing me, he was unable to work. Also he couldn't sleep but a few hours and his appetite was poor. Antidepressant medication and relaxation training, using a combination of hypnotic and meditation approaches, were used along with psychotherapy.

In therapy his religious beliefs were also explored. As part of an educational approach, the ideas about religious fanaticism and mature spirituality were presented as an idea for him to consider. He recognized very quickly that his parents had brought him up on the fanatical side of religion. He moved away from it when he was healthy and enjoyed life in moderation. However, under stress, he tended to fall back on fanatic religiosity which in its turn made him more obsessed with guilt and damnation, leading to severe depression and anxiety.

He became very much interested in learning more about these matters, and we discussed it in some detail. He also read the books I recommended (books by Rollo May, Thomas Merton, Scott Peck, and Eric Fromm). His symptoms improved quickly once he got an understanding of his problem, which he had been told before by many was just a chemical inbalance. His "manic depressive illness" improved dramatically in a few months. He continued to work on changing his compulsive personality. After some ups and downs in their relationship, his wife also became more flexible; and their relationship became much better. Since then he has been living a healthy life emotionally and spiritually sans the old guilt trips. His old monster God was replaced by an understanding, compassionate, and fair God. He moved from excessive rigidity and perfectionism to healthy discipline. As it turned out, there are more ways than one to balance the chemical inbalance.

Flip-Floppers. Several individuals that I have been able to help with the ideas in this book are people who used to go back and forth between fanatic religion, antireligion, or no religion. They all had backgrounds of rigid moralistic families where the parents preached fanatical religion and practiced hypocrisy (as the children saw it). In some cases the parents, or one of the parents, had insisted on the child being a strict adherent to a particular denomination. In at least one case, the situation had gone even further and the parent convinced the child that everybody except those belonging to a particular local church would go to Hell. As these children grew up, they found it intellectually dishonest and spiritually wrong to follow the example of the parents. So, they would move to an antireligous or areligious stance and pursue that for awhile. The dissatisfactions of spiritual needs and the fears instilled during childhood would slowly catch up with them. At such times, emotionally scared and spiritually hungry, they would try the religion of their parents for a while. At first, they would feel some relief and release of tensions and new hope. But that would gradually fade; and they would get really unhappy and move from the confusion back to the areligious phase. For them, religion was either their parents' type or nothing.

As I explored their experiences and explained the possibility of a quite different kind of spiritual experience and life, they were eager to learn more. As they learned more, they made important changes to become genuinely spiritually healthy, becoming more open, courageous, and loving. Those changes stopped their flip-flopping in the religious sphere and helped them also to eliminate confusion and instability in other aspects of life.

A Case of Physical and Moral Hypochondria. Jim was in his late thirties when he started seeing me for treatment of hypochondriasis. He was afraid that he was developing colon cancer. He used to check for evidences of bleeding everytime after he used the toilet. Even after two separate specialists did extensive workups and assured Jim that he had no colon cancer, he continued to be preoccupied with it.

Some of his relatives had colon problems including cancer in the case of one person. Interestingly enough, Jim had also what may be called moral hypochondriasis, a pervasive sense of sinfulness without real reason. The role spiritual issues played in Jim's illness and in the way his spiritual and physical health improved are illustrative of many of the points I have made in preceding chapters.

Jim grew up in an orthodox Catholic family. His parents— particularly his mother—were quite negative in their thinking. Their approach to life was one of excessive guilt over past mistakes and high levels of anxiety regarding mistakes they may make in the future. Jim learned a highly critical (judgmental) attitude from his parents and applied it to himself and others.

Although Jim had hypochondriacal tendencies (tendency to exaggerate physical symptoms and worry about them), his problem came to a head only when he was going through a spiritual crisis. Growing up among Christian Fundamentalists (some of whom would fit the description of fanatics), Jim had some doubts about his liberal Catholic faith off and on. About a year prior to coming to see me, Jim was repeatedly confronted by a group of Christian Fundamentalist friends about the issues of death and salvation. This shook up Jim's faith and he started having serious doubts about his spirituality. For a while he thought of joining the fundamentalistic-fanatic group. However, something deep down kept telling him to look carefully at the shallowness, hypocrisy, and hatefulness of these friends who were preaching Christian love and goodness. In fact, Jim's intellectual honesty so turned him off against religious fanatics that he went through a phase of being atheistic and areligious prior to his symptoms coming to a head.

As Jim's conflict over religion got worse, so did his hypochondriasis. Then he joined a healthy prayer group. This group consisted of several people who were open minded, genuinely loving, and integrated. The healthy spirituality of these friends was quite attractive to Jim, but his doubts and fears stimulated by the fanatics continued to haunt him.

It was at such a time of conflict and intensified symptoms of hypochondriasis that Jim first saw me. As I explored his fears, it was clear that the fear of death and damnation was at the root of his anxiety. Explorations of his guilt showed it was neurotic guilt. Jim was flip-flopping between healthy and unhealthy aspects of religion for a while. We analyzed the psychological factors behind both sides of his religious life.

The unhealthy aspects of Jim's spirituality showed the following elements: excessive fears about God, damnation, intellectual doubts, search for truth, love for people of other faiths and so on. His fanatic side told him to be rigid, exclusive in his identity and love, and to keep his mind closed around the tenets of hyperfundamentalism.

Excessive Guilt. Jim was a perfectionist and felt guilty about falling short of expectations. He felt terribly guilty about even small mistakes. His guilt had underlying fear of God's wrath and punishment rather than regret for breaking the principles of love.

Self-Hate: Jim's self-hate started as a child—based on the negative feedback he got from his parents. His religion reinforced it by making him feel like a terrible sinner.

Hate of Others: Jim was hateful to those people who were different from himself. He would get furious about their laziness, superficiality, ungodliness, and so on. His only daughter, who was very insecure and appeared lazy, was a victim of Jim's hate.

Closedminded: The fanatical part of Jim wanted to cling to some simplistic ideas and to reject the urge to search for truth. Also, doubts were repressed and intuitive abilities shut out.

Need for Control: Jim had a strong need to be in control of himself and people around him. Therefore Jim was uptight and tense. He tried to control other people by moralizing, guilt trips on them, and use of scare tactics (hellfire) and shame.

The healthy side of Jim's spirituality showed the following features:
Openness of Vision and Search for Truth: Jim read some good books on spirituality while he was apparently on the healthy side of spirituality. He used his doubts to explore spiritual and psychological aspects of life deeply. He was quite open to exploring spiritual conflicts in therapy.

Love: Jim's healthy side had genuine love of himself, others, and God. This God was a loving God who genuinely cared for everybody's welfare. Jim was understanding, nurturing, and willing to sacrifice selfish interests when he was on the healthy side of spirituality. He loved himself as a human being and as a special individual.

Courage: The healthy side of Jim showed courage to face difficulties and pain, doubts and the uncertainties of life. It also helped his search for truth.

Prudence: When his healthy side had the upper hand, Jim was cautious not to jump to conclusions or leap into important actions before careful consideration of consequences.
These two sides of Jim went on flip/flopping until he realized what was happening. Once he realized the psychological factors behind his two opposing religious tendencies, he chose to reinforce the healthy side. It took considerable effort and many ups and downs before he could bring about the change. His hypochondriasis, both physical and moral, has cleared almost completely.

Approaches in Spiritual Growth: In all these and other cases of spiritual growth, there are three important approaches:

1. *Exploration of one's own faith and improving knowledge:* The Socratic dictum "an unexamined life is not worth living" is particularly true of one's faith. In the above cases, individuals were willing to examine their faith and its effect on their lives. As they explored, they gradually recognized how their religion was making them scared, hateful, narrowminded, and the like rather than loving, courageous, prudent, and wise. So these people looked for better alternatives—new outlooks. Simultaneously they also worked on overcoming neurotic fears and facing existential anxiety.

2. *Facing fears:* All these individuals had neurotic fears because of their religious beliefs. Also, they had not properly faced the existential issues. Moreover, all of them had varying degrees of fear about examining their faith. Therefore, it was a slow process with backsliding from time to time. But as they faced the fears, they could see the benefit of overcoming fears and that encouraged further search.

3. *Growing in love:* Varying degrees of self-hate—and hate of others—was part of the problem. Some of them equated self-love with the sin of pride. As they learned more about love as opposed to hate, or of pride and greed, they were able to become genuinely loving. Also with more courage, they could take the risk of loving themselves and others.

With these changes their identity broadened, became stronger and more inclusive. They could face their shadow or negative aspect and integrate it into a healthy wholeness. Previously they blocked it out of awareness or projected it onto others.

Good reading, reflection, meditations, prayer, open discussion with the therapist, and attending spiritual workshops were some of the most important practical steps taken. Some individuals also joined spiritual study groups.

CONCLUSION

"Authentic religion is the clearest opening through which the inexhaustible energies of the cosmos can pour into human existence."[1] [Huston Smith]

In many ways we live in the best of times and the worst of times. Never before have so many people lived so comfortably for so long. And never before have human beings been so close to total destruction of themselves and their environment by their own sweet hands. The forces of good and of evil seem to have reached the zenith at this point in history.

Even as the world is spending more on weapons than ever before, the efforts for peace are growing strong. Even as conformism and rebellion are vastly evident, authenticity is showing vitality and vigor. In spite of widespread dichotomous thinking, holistic understanding is gaining ground. Psychological mindedness and depth are fighting against mechanical thinking and superficiality. As the world is shrinking to a global village and the private world of the individual is ever expanding, an increasing number of individuals are transcending their cultural barriers and gaining a universal sense of identity.

We are caught between the dusk of a passing age and the dawn of a hopefully better era. The cross-currents of vast change are causing insecurity, confusion in belief and sense of belonging, and hurt pride in many individuals and groups. Many others are suffering from the consequences of excessive power and glory. These negative effects are causing defensive and offensive reactions of fundamentalistic rigidities and fanatic destructiveness.

Religion is supposed to fight evil and promote goodness. However (in reality) religion itself is a battleground—perhaps the biggest battleground—between the forces of good and evil. On one side are the forces of healthy spirituality, and on the other the forces of unhealthy religiosity. Because of this internal conflict, religion behaves like a massive multiple personality with an enormous Dr. Jekyll and an equally huge Mr. Hyde unceremoniously welded together into a confounding whole.

As we have seen in the preceding chapters, the dynamic factors in healthy spirituality are love, wisdom, courage, and prudence. Not surprisngly, these are also the elments in the dynamics of goodness. *These factors are intimately interinked with healthy identity and integration*—a crucial fact often overlooked, unfortunately. The opposite elements are involved in unhealthy religiosity as well as in the dynamics of evil.

Spiritually healthy influences have been gaining strength in religions—as evidenced by efforts for peace and justice, consciousness raising, authenticity, integration and ecumenism. The spirit of ecumenism was beautifully expressed on two occasions during the Fall of 1986 at Assisi, Italy. In the first instance, representatives of various world religions met under the auspices of the World Wild Life Fund for promoting conservation of nature, and the second ecumenical gathering organized by Pope John Paul II was hailed by many as a spiritual summit. Assisi—famous for the 13th century friar St. Francis of Assisi, who was a lover of nature and strong proponent of love and peace—was indeed an appropriate site for these meetings. Although the Pope was acting in the best Christian spirit to enhance love and peace, Christian extremists condemned his move—one even characterized the meeting as the "greatest single abomination in church history."

Religious fundamentalism—and fanaticism along with it—has been gaining strength in different parts of the world in the past decade. Christian fundamentalism in the United States, Islamic, Jewish and Christian fundamentalism in the Middle East, and Hindu, Sikh and Islamic fundamentalism in India are examples. Our explorations in the previous chapters have shown that fundamentalism/fanaticism are not simply matters of hypocrisy as many people think, but much more complex.

Understanding the complex dynamics of the healthy and unhealthy aspects of religion enables us to make the right choices and move along the proper path of spiritual growth. And, as we saw, spiritual growth is holistic growth—development of the total person. It is exactly opposite to the cancerous growth of one part at the expense of the whole. Healing at the Temple of Asklepios in Greece involved treatment of the whole person—including physical, psychological, social, and religious aspects—indicating the wisdom of a holistic approach.

When the pure light of spirituality emanating from the mystical source passes through the prism of human experience, it transforms into a spectrum of radiant religious colors. Each color has its own beauty, but the more it distances itself from the source of light and tries to be exclusive, the deeper it falls into the darkness of unhealthy religiosity.

It is often said that we live in an age of crisis. The Chinese ideogram for crisis indicates problems as well as opportunities. As we face immense problems, we also have the benefit of the accumulated wisdom of science and religion. That wisdom can help us to actualize our individual and collective potential for growth and prevent our propensity for destruction. The challenge has never been greater, nor the opportunity more profound.

APPENDIX

Psychological Defense Mechanisms

Classification According to George E. Vaillant in *Adaptation To Life* (Boston: Little Brown & Company, 1977, p. 80).

Psychotic Mechanisms (common in psychosis, dreams, and childhood)
Denial (of external reality)
Distortion
Delusional Projection

Immature Mechanisms (common in severe depression, personality disorders, and adolescence)
Fantasy (schizoid withdrawal, denial through fantasy)
Projection
Hypochondriasis
Passive-Aggressive Behavior (masochism, turning against the self)
Acting Out (compulsive delinquency, perversion)

Neurotic Mechanisms (common in everyone)
Intellectualization (isolation, obsessive behavior, undoing, rationalization)
Repression
Reaction Formation
Displacement (conversion, phobias, wit)
Dissociation (neurotic denial)

Mature Mechanisms (common in "healthy" adults)
Sublimation
Altruism
Suppression
Anticipation
Humor

Altruism is active regard for the interests and needs of others.

Sublimation is a substitute activity that meets instinctual needs.

Suppression is consciously inhibiting an impulse (Repression is an unconscious process.)

Anticipation involves healthy planning for the future.

ENDNOTES

Introduction

[1]Arnold Toynbee, *An Historian's Approach to Religion* (London: Oxford University Press, 1956), pp. 286 & 287.

Chapter 2

[1]H. G. Wells, *The Outline of History* (New York: Doubleday & Company, Inc., 1971), p. 568.

[2]Ibid., p. 339.

[3]Mark Twain, *Letters From the Earth* (New York: Perennial Library, Harper & Row, Publishers, 1962), p. 180.

[4]Herbert Spiegel and David Spiegel, *Trance and Treatment* (New York: Basic Books, Inc. Publishers, 1978), p. 125.

Chapter 3

[1]Rabindranath Tagore, *The Collected Poems and Plays of Rabindranath Tagore* (New York: Macmillan Publishing Co., Inc., 1937), p. 13.

[2]Ibid., p. 27.

[3]Martin Buber, *Good and Evil* (New York: Charles Scribner's Sons, 1952), p. 97.

[4]Kahlil Gibran, *The Prophet* (New York: Alfred A. Knopf, 1982), p. 50.

[5]Wallace B. Clift, *Jung and Christianity* (New York: Crossroad Publishing Company, 1983), p. 105.

[6]Viktor E. Frankl, *The Unconscious God* (New York: Simon & Schuster, Inc., 1975), p. 28.

[7]Paul Tillich, *Dynamic of Faith* (New York: Harper & Row, Publishers, 1957), p. 105.

[8]Hazrat Inayat Khan, *Spiritual Dimensions of Psychology* (New York: Sufi Order Publications, 1981), p. 50.

[9]Thomas Merton, *Contemplation In a World of Action* (New York: Doubleday and Company, Inc.: Image Books, 1973), p. 231.

[10]Thomas Merton, *The Way of Chuang Tzu* (New York: New Directions Publishing Corporation, 1969), p. 83.

[11]Radhakrishnan, *Selected Writings on Philosophy, Religion, and Culture.* Edited by Robert A. McDermott (New York: E. P. Dutton & Company, Inc., 1970) p. 53.

Chapter 4

[1]William James, *The Varieties of Religious Experience* (New York: The New American Library, Inc., 1958), p. 265.

[2]Erich Fromm, *Marx's Concept of Man* (New York: Frederick Unger Publishing Co., 1966), p. 44

[3]Rollo May, *Freedom and Destiny* (New York: W. W. Norton & Company, 1981), pp. 199-200.

[4]Ibid., p. 202.

[5]Boris Pasternak, *Dr. Zhivago,* trans. Bernard Guilbert Guerney (New York: Signet Books, 1958), p. 44.

[6]Erich Fromm, *Psychoanalysis and Religion* (New Haven: Yale University Press, 1950) p. 108.

[7]William James, *The Varieties of Religious Experience* (New York: The New American Library, Inc., 1958), p. 267.

[8]Joseph Fletcher, *Situation Ethics: The New Morality* (Philadelphia: West Minster Press, n.d.), p. 17.

Chapter 5

[1]Bertrand Russell, *Why I am Not a Christian* (New York: Simon & Schuster, Inc., 1957), p. 24.

[2]Raja Rao, Professor of Religion at the University of Texas and writer (Personal Communications).

[3]Leo Tolstoi, *The Works of Leo Tolstoi* (New York: Walter J. Black, Inc., n.d.), p. 162.

[4]Thomas Merton, *Love and Living*, ed. Naomi Burton Stone and Brother Patrick Hart (New York: Farrar, Straus and Giroux, 1980), p. 92.

[5]Walter Kaufman, ed., *Existentialism from Dostoevsky to Sartre* (New York: The New American Library, Inc., 1975), p. 378.

[6]Rollo May, *Freedom and Destiny* (New York: W. W. Norton & Company, 1981), p. 89.

[7]Ibid., p. 169.

[8]Fyodor Dostoevsky, *The Brothers Karamazov* (New York: Bantam Books, Inc., 1971), p. 309.

[9]J. M. Nouwen, *Reaching Out* (New York: Doubleday & Company, Inc., 1975), p. 30.

[10]Paul Tillich, *The Courage To Be* (New Haven: Yale University Press, 1952), p. 77.

Chapter 6

[1]Erich Fromm, *Greatness and Limitations of Freud's Thought* (New York: New American Library, 1980), p. 48.

[2]Alexander Lowen, M. D., *Narcissism* (New York: Macmillan Publishing Co., Inc., 1983), p. 75.

[3]Sigmund Freud, *Group Psychology and the Analysis of the Ego* (New York: W. W. Norton & Company, 1959), p. 66.

[4]Erich Fromm, *The Heart of Man* (New York: Harper & Row, Publishers, 1964), pp. 81-82.

[5]Quoted by Thomas Merton in *The Nonviolent Alternatives* (New York: Farrar, Straus, Giroux, 1971), p. 214.

[6]Reinhold Niebuhr, *The Nature and Destiny of Man* (New York: Scribner's, 1949), p. 213.

[7]Ibid., p. 214.

Chapter 7

[1]Teilhard de Chardin, *The Phenomenon of Man* (New York: Harper & Row, Publishers, 1959), p. 265.

[2]Erich Fromm, *The Art of Loving* (New York: Harper & Row, Publishers, 1956), p. 22.

[3]M. Scott Peck, M.D., *The Road Less Traveled* (New York: Simon & Schuster, Inc., 1978), p. 81.

[4]William Johnston, *The Inner Eye of Love* (San Francisco: Harper & Row, Publishers, 1978), p. 65.

Chapter 8

[1]Jerome D. Frank, Ph.D., M.D., *Sanity and Survival in the Nuclear Age* (New York: Random House, 1982), p. 134.

[2]Charles A. Pinderhughes, "Differential Bonding: Toward a Psychophysiological Theory of Stereotyping," *The American Journal of Psychiatry*, January, 1979, pp. 33-37.

[3]James M. Washington (editors), *A Testament of Hope* (New York, Harper and Row, 1986), p. 290.

[4]Sam Keen, *Faces of the Enemy* (Harper & Row, San Francisco, 1986), p. 172.

[5]Jerome D. Frank, Ph.D., M.D., *Sanity and Survival in the Nuclear Age* (New York: Random House, 1982), pp. 131-132.

[6]Grace Halsell, *Prophecy and Politics* (West Port, CT: Lawrence Hill & Co., 1986), p. 116.

Chapter 9

[1]Steven F. Brena, M.D., *Yoga and Medicine* (New York: The Julian Press, 1972), p. 169.

[2]Dermot Cox, O. F. M., *The Trimuph of Impotence* (Rome: University Gregoriana Editrice, 1978), p. 176.

[3]Abraham Joshua Heschel, *A Passion for Truth* (New York: Farrar, Strauss & Giroux 1973), p. 297.

[4]Paul Tillich, *The New Being* (New York: Charles Scribner's Sons, n.d.), p. 68.

[5]Gordon W. Allport, *The Nature of Prejudice* (New York: Doubleday & Company, 1958), p. 415.

[6]Edward K. Braxton, *The Wisdom Community* (New York: Paulist Press, 1980), p. 185.

[7]Lawrence Kohlberg, *The Philosophy of Moral Development* (San Francisco: Harper & Row, Publishers, 1981), pp. 409-412.

[8]Fritjof Capra, *The Tao of Physics* (Boston: New Science Library, Shambhala Publications, Inc., 1983), p. 305.

[9]Paul Tillich, *The Eternal Now* (New York: Charles Scribner's Sons, 1964), p. 167.

[10]John A. Sanford, *The Kingdom Within* (New York: Paulist Press, 1970).

Chapter 10

[1]Robert A. McDermott, ed., *Radhakrishnan* (New York: E. P. Dutton & Company, Inc., 1970), p. 136.

[2]Ibid., p. 137.

[3]Erik H. Erikson, *Dimensions of a New Identity* (New York: W. W. Norton & Company, 1974), pp. 27-28.

[4]Erik H. Erikson, *Identity Youth and Crisis* (New York: W. W. Norton & Company, 1968), pp. 80-81.

[5]Erik H. Erikson, *Dimensions of a New Identity* (New York: W. W. Norton & Company, 1974), p. 28.

[6]Hans Mol, *Identity and the Sacred* (New York: The Free Press, 1976), p. 6.

[7]Dobson, Hindson, Falwell, *The Fundamentalist Phenomenon* (Grand Rapids: Baker House Books, 1986), p. 147.

[8]Albert Nolan, *Jesus Before Christianity* (New York: Orbis Books, 1978), pp. 118-119.

[9]Aldous Huxley in introduction to *The Song of God: Bhagavad-Gita,* translated by Swami Prabhavananda and Christopher Isherwood (New York: The New American Library, Inc., 1972), p. 13.

[10]Rollo May, *The Discovery of Being* (New York: W. W. Norton & Company, 1983), p. 102.

Chapter 11

[1]Elena Malits ,"Thomas Merton and the Possibilities of Religious Imagination", in *The Message of Thomas Merton,* edited by Brother Patrick Hart (Cistercian Publications, Kalamazoo, 1981).

[2]Michael Mott, *The Seven Mountains of Thomas Merton* (Boston: Houghton Mifflin Company, 1984), p. 443.

[3]*The Asian Journal of Thomas Merton,* Edited from his original notebooks by Naomi Burton, Brother Patrick Hart and James Laughlin (New York: NewDirectionsPublishing Corporation, 1975), p. 235.

[4]Paul Wilkes, ed., *Merton by Those Who Knew Him Best* (San Francisco: Harper & Row, Publishers, 1984), p. 7.

[5]Deba Patnaik, ed., *A Merton Concelebration* (Notre Dame, Indiana: Ave Maria Press, 1981), p. 16.

[6]Thomas Merton, *Love and Living,* ed. Naomi Burton Stone and Brother Patrick Hart (New York: Farrar, Straus and Giroux, 1979), Chapter One.

[7]Ibid., p. 25.

[8]Ibid., p. 25.

[9]Ibid., p. 25.

[10]Ibid., p. 25.

[11]Ibid., p. 31

[12]Mathew Fox, *Breakthrough: Meister Eckhart's Creation Spirituality* in new translation (New York: Doubleday & Co. 1980).

[13]Monica Furlong, *Merton: A Biography* (New York: Bantam Books, Inc., 1981), p. 78.

Chapter 12

[1]Thomas Merton, *The Nonviolent Alternative* (New York: Farrar, Straus and Giroux, 1980), p. 180.

[2]James Michaels, "Two Days That Shook the World," *India Abroad,* January 27, 1984.

[3]William Johnston, *The Inner Eye of Love* (San Francisco: Harper & Row, Publishers, 1978), p. 26.

[4]Louis Fischer, *Gandhi* (New York: The New American Library, Inc., 1954), pp. 142-143.

[5]Erik H. Erikson, *Gandhi's Truth* (New York: W. W. Norton & Company, 1969), p. 403.

[6]Ibid., p. 405.

Chapter 13

[1]Delos Banning McKown, *With Faith and Fury* (Buffalo, New York: Prometheus Books, 1985), p. 438.

Chapter 14

[1]Shiva Naipaul, *Journey To Nowhere: A New World Tragedy* (New York: Simon & Schuster, Inc., 1981), p. 297.

Conclusion

[1]Huston Smith, *The Religions of Man* (New York: Harper & Row, Publishers, 1958), p. 11.

BIBLIOGRAPHY

Adler, Mortimer J., *Six Great Ideas* (New York: Macmillan Publishing Co., Inc., 1981).

Appel, Willa, *Cults in America* (New York: Holt, Reinhart and Winston, 1983).

Allport, Gordon W., *The Individual and His Religion* (New York: Macmillan Publishing Co., Inc., 1950).

Allport, Gordon W., *The Nature of Prejudice* (New York: Doubleday & Company, Inc., 1958).

Arestah, Reza A., *Final Integration In the Adult Personality* (Leiden, Netherlands: E. J. Brill, 1965).

Barnhouse, Ruth Tiffany, *Identity* (Philadelphia: The Westminster Press, 1984).

Baum, Gregory, *Religion and Alienation* (New York: Paulist Press, 1975).

Becker, Ernest, *Escape From Evil* (New York: The Free Press, 1975).

Braxton, Edward K., *The Wisdom Community* (New York: Paulist Press, 1980).

Brena, Steven F., M.D., *Yoga and Medicine* (New York: The Julian Press, 1972).

Brown, L. B., ed., *Advances in the Psychology of Religion* (Oxford: Pergamon Press, 1985).

Bruteau, Beatrice, *Contemplative Review* (Barre, Vermont: Fall, 1983).

Buber, Martin, *Good and Evil* (New York: Charles Scribner's Sons, 1952).

Byrnes, Joseph F., *The Psychology of Religion* (New York: The Free Press, 1984).

Capra, Fritjof, *The Tao of Physics* (Boston: Shambhala Publications, Inc., 1983).

Clift, Wallace B., *Jung and Christianity* (New York: Crossroad Publishing Company, 1983).

Cox, Dermot, O. F. M., *The Triumph of Impotence* (Roma: Universita Gregoriana Editrice, 1978).

Cox, Harvey, *Religion in the Secular City* (New York: Simon & Schuster, Inc., 1984).

de Chardin, Teilhard, *The Phenomenon of Man* (New York: Harper & Row, Publishers, 1959).

Dodson, Hindson, Falwell, *The Fundamentalist Phenomenon* (Grand Rapids, Michigan: Baker House Books, 1986).

Dostoevsky, Fyodor, *The Brothers Karamazov* (New York: Bantam Books Inc., 1971).

Easwaran, Eknath, *Gandhi: The Man* (Petaluma, California: Nilgiri Press, 1978).

Erikson, Erik H., *Gandhi's Truth* (New York: W. W. Norton & Company, 1969).

Erikson, Erik H., *Dimensions of a New Identity* (New York: W. W. Norton & Company, 1974).

Erikson, Erik H., *Identity Youth and Crisis* (New York: W. W. Norton & Company, 1974).

Fischer, Louis, *Gandhi* (New York: The New American Library, Inc., 1954).

Fletcher, Joseph, *Situation Ethics: The New Morality* (Philadelphia: Westminster Press, n.d.).

Fowler, James, *Stages of Faith* (San Francisco: Harper & Row Publishers, 1981).

Fox, Matthew, *Breakthrough: Meister Eckhart's Creation Spirituality in New Translation* (New York: Doubleday & Co. 1980).

Fox, Matthew, *Compassion* (Minneapolis, Minnesota: Winston Press, 1979).

Frank, Jerome D., Ph.D., M.D., *Sanity and Survival in the Nuclear Age* (New York: Random House, 1982).

Frankl, Viktor E., *The Unconscious God* (New York: Washington Square Press, 1975).

Freud, Sigmund, *Civilization and its Discontents* (New York: W. W. Norton & Company, 1960).

Freud, Sigmund, *Group Psychology & the Analysis of the Ego* (New York: W. W. Norton & Company, 1959).

Freud, Sigmund, *The Future of an Illusion* (New York: W. W. Norton & Company, 1961).

Fromm, Erich, *Marx's Concept of Man* (New York: Frederick Unger Publishing Co., Inc., 1966).

Fromm, Erich, *The Heart of Man* (New York: Harper & Row, Publishers, 1964).

Fromm, Erich, *The Art of Loving* (New York: Harper & Row, Publishers, 1956).

Fromm, Erich, *Greatness and Limitations of Freud's Thought* (New York: Mentor Books, 1980).

Fromm, Erich, *To Have or to Be* (New York: Bantam Books, Inc., 1981).

Fromm, Erich, *Psychoanalysis and Religion* (New Haven: Yale University Press, 1950).

Fromm, Erich, *The Anatomy of Human Destructiveness* (New York: Fawcett Crest, 1973).

Fromm, Erich, *Zen Buddhism and Psychoanalysis* (New York: Harper & Row, 1960).

Furlong, Monica, *Merton: A Biography* (New York: Bantam Books, Inc., 1981).

Galanter, Marc, "Charismatic Religious Sects and Psychiatry: An Overview," *American Journal of Psychiatry*, December 1982, Vol. 134, No. 12.

Gandhi, M. K., *An Autobiography* (New York: Penguin Books, 1982).

Gibran, Kahlil, *The Prophet* (New York: Alfred A. Knopf, 1982).

Goleman, Daniel, *Vital Lies, Simple Truths* (New York: Simon & Schuster, Inc. 1985).

Halperin, David A., ed., *Religion, Sect and Cult* (Boston: John Wright Publishing Co., 1983).

Halsell, Grace, *Prophecy and Politics* (Westport, CT: Lawrence Hill & Co., 1986).

Hazrat, Inayat Khan, *Spiritual Dimensions of Psychology* (New York: Sufi Order Publications, 1981).

Heschel, Abraham Joshua, *A Passion For Truth* (New York: Farrar, Straus & Giroux, 1973).

Hoffer, Eric, *The True Believer* (New York: Harper & Row, Publishers, 1951).

James, William, *The Varieties of Religious Experience* (New York: The New American Library, Inc., 1958).

Johnston, William, *The Inner Eye of Love* (San Francisco: Harper & Row, Publishers, 1978).

Jung, Carl Gustav, *Psychology and the East* (Princeton University Press, 1978).

Jung, Carl Gustav, *Psychology and Western Religion* (Princeton University Press, 1984).

Jung, Carl Gustav, *Modern Man in Search of a Soul* (New York: Harcourt Brace Jovanovich, 1933).

Kaufman, Walter, ed., *Existentialism From Dostoevsky to Sartre* (New York: The New American Library, Inc., 1975).

Keen, Sam, *Faces of the Enemy* (San Francisco: Harper & Row, 1986).

Kerns, Wead, *People's Temple—People's Tomb* (Plainfield, NJ: Logos International, 1979).

Kilduff, Jabers, *The Suicide Cult* (New York: Bantam, 1978).

Kohlberg, Lawrence, *The Philosophy of Moral Development* (San Francisco: Harper and Row, 1981).

Krause, Stern, *Guyana Massacre* (New York: Berkeley Pub. Co., 1978).

Kung, Hans, *Freud and the Problem of God* (New Haven: Yale University Press, 1979).

Lasch, Christopher, *Culture of Narcissism* (New York: W. W. Norton & Company, 1978).

Laurer, Jeanette, and Robert Laurer, "Marriages Made to Last," in *Psychology Today* (Washington, DC, June 1985).

Lewis, Sinclair, *Elmer Gantry* (New York: The New American Library, 1970).

Levine, Saul V., "Cults and Mental Health: Clinical Conclusions," *Canadian Journal of Psychiatry,* December, 1981.

Levine, Saul V., M.D., *Radical Departures* (San Diego: Harcourt, Brace, Jovanovich, Publishers, 1984).

Liddy, Gordon G., *Will* (New York: St. Martin's Press, 1980).

Lovinger, Robert J., *Working With Religious Issues In Therapy,* (New York: Jason Arson, Inc., 1984).

Lowen, Alexander, M.D., *Narcissism* (New York: Macmillan Publishing Co., Inc., 1983).

Marsden, George M., *Fundamentalism and American Culture* (New York: Oxford University Press, 1982).

Maslow, Abraham H., *Religions, Values, and Peak-Experiences* (New York: Penguin Books, 1978).

Maslow, Abraham H., *Toward a Psychology of Being* (New York: D. Van Nostrand Company, 1968).

May, Rollo, *The Discovery of Being* (New York: W. W. Norton & Company, 1983).

May, Rollo, *Freedom and Destiny* (New York: W. W. Norton and Company, 1981)

May, Rollo, *Man's Search for Himself* (New York: W. W. Norton and Company, 1953).

McKown, Delos Banning, *With Faith and Fury* (Buffalo, New York: Prometheus Books, 1985).

Menninger, Karl, *Whatever Became of Sin* (New York: Bantam Books, 1978).

Merton, Thomas, *Contemplation in a World of Action* (New York: Image Books, Doubleday & Company, 1973).

Merton, Thomas, *Gandhi on Non-Violence* (New York: New Directions Publishing Corporation, 1965).

Merton, Thomas, *New Seeds of Contemplation* (New York: New Directions Publishing Corporation, 1961).

Merton, Thomas, *The Asian Journal of Thomas Merton* ed. Naomi Burton, Brother Patrick Hart and James Laughlin, (New York: New Directions Publishing Corporation, 1973).

Merton, Thomas, *The Nonviolent Alternative* (New York: Farrar, Straus and Giroux, 1980).

Merton, Thomas, *The Way of Chuang Tzu* (New York: New Directions Publishing Corporation, 1969).

Merton, Thomas, *Love and Living,* ed. Naomi Burton Stone and Brother Patrick Hart (New York: Farrar, Straus and Giroux, 1980).

Merton, Thomas, *The Seven Storey Mountain* (New York: Harcourt Brace Jovanovich, Publishers, 1948).

Michaels, James, "Two Days That Shook the World," *India Abroad,* New York, 27 January 1984.

Moody, Raymond, *Life After Life* (New York: Bantam Books, 1975).

Mott, Michael, *The Seven Mountains of Thomas Merton* (Boston: Houghton Mifflin Company, 1984).

Naipaul, Shiva, *Journey to Nowhere: A New World Tragedy* (New York: Simon & Schuster, Inc., 1981).

Niebuhr, Reinhold, *The Nature and Destiny of Man* (New York: Scribner's, 1949).

Nouwen, Henri J. M., *Reaching Out* (New York: Doubleday & Company, Inc., 1971).

Oates, Wayne, *When Religion Gets Sick* (Philadelphia: The Westminster Press, n.d.).

Pasternak, Boris, *Doctor Zhivago* (New York: The New American Library, 1958).

Patnaik, Deba, ed., *A Merton Concelebration* (Notre Dame, Indiana: Ave Mari Press, 1981).

Peck, M. Scott, *People of the Lie* (New York: Simon & Schuster, Inc., 1983).

Peck, M. Scott, *The Road Less Traveled* (New York: Simon & Schuster, Inc., 1978).

Pinderhughes, Charles, "Differential Bonding: Toward a Psychophysiological Theory of Stereotyping," *The American Journal of Psychiatry*, January 1979.

Radhakrishnan, *Recovery of Faith* (New York: Harper Brother Publishers, n.d.).

Radhakrishnan, *Selected Writings on Philosophy, Religion, and Culture* (New York: E. P. Dutton & Company, Inc., 1970), ed. by Robert A. McDermott.

Robinson, Lillian H., ed., *Psychiatry and Religion: Overlapping Concerns* (Washington: American Psychiatric Press, 1986).

Rokeach, Milton, *The Open and Closed Mind* (New York: Basic Books, 1960).

Rubin, Theodore I., *One to One* (New York: Viking Press, 1983).

Rubin, Theodore I., *Compassion and Self-Hate* (New York: Ballantine Books, 1982).

Russell, Bertrand, *Why I Am Not a Christian* (New York: Simon & Schuster, Inc., 1957).

Samford, John A., *Evil* (New York: Crossroad Publishing Company, 1982).

Samford, John A., *The Kingdom Within* (New York: Paulist Press, 1970).

Sartre, Jean Paul, "Portrait of the Antisemite," in *Existentialism from Dostoevsky to Sartre*, ed. Walter Kaufman, (New York: The New American Library, Inc., 1979).

Skinner, B. F., *Beyond Freedom and Dignity* (New York: Alfred A. Knopf, Inc., 1971).

Smith, Huston, *The Religions of Man* (New York: Harper & Row, Publishers, 1958).

Spiegel, Herbert, and David Spiegel, *Trance & Treatment* (New York: Basic Books, 1978).

Storr, Anthony, *Human Aggression* (New York: Bantam Books, 1970).

Tagore, Rabindranath, *The Collected Poems & Plays of Rabindranath Tagore* (New York: Macmillan Publishing Co., Inc., 1949).

Tillich, Paul, *Dynamics of Faith* (New York: Harper & Row, Publishers, 1957).

Tillich, Paul, *The Courage to Be* (New Haven: Yale University Press, 1952).

Tillich, Paul, *The Eternal Now* (New York: Charles Scribner's Sons, 1963).

Tillich, Paul, *The New Being* (New York: Charles Scribner's Sons, 1955).

Tolstoi, Leo, "The Death of Ivan Ilyitch," in *The Works of Leo Tolstoi* (New York: Walter J. Black, Inc., 1923).

Toynbee, Arnold, *An Historian's Apporach to Religion* (London: Oxford University Press, 1956).

Twain, Mark, *Letters from the Earth* (New York: Harper & Row, Publishers, 1962).

Washington, James M., ed., *A Testament of Hope* (New York: Harper & Row, 1986).

Wells, H. G., *The Outline of History* (New York: Doubleday & Company, Inc., 1971).

Wilkes, Paul, ed., *Merton by Those Who Knew Him Best* (San Francisco: Harper & Row, Publishers, 1984).

Yalom, Irvin D., *Existential Psychotherapy* (New York: Basic Books, 1980).

Permissions

Permission to reprint from the following material is gratefully acknowledged to the holders of copyright:

From Kahlil Gibran's *The Prophet*, by permission of Alfred A. Knopf, Inc., New York, N.Y. Copyright 1923 by Kahlil Gibran and renewed 1951 by Administrators C.T.A. of Kahlil Gibran Estate, and Mary G. Gibran.

From Rabindranath Tagore's *Gitanjali*, (New York: Macmillan, 1913), by permission of Macmillan Publishing Company, a division of Macmillan, Inc., New York, N.Y.

From Thomas Merton's *The Way of Chuang Tzu*, copyright 1965 by The Abbey of Gethsemani, by permission of New Directions Publishing Co., New York, N.Y.

From *The Song of God: Bhagavad-Tita*, translated by Swami Prabhavananda and Christopher Isherwood, copyright 1972, by permission of Vedanta Press, Hollywood, California.

From George E. Vaillant's *Adaptations to Life*, copyright 1977 by George E. Vaillant, by permission of Little, Brown and Company, Boston, Massachusetts.

From Rollo May's *The Discovery of Being*, copyright 1983, by permission of W. W. Norton & Co., Inc., New York, N.Y.

From Erik H. Erikson's *Dimensions of a New Identity*, copyright 1974, and from his *Identity, Youth and Crisis*, copyright 1968, by permission of W. W. Norton & Co., Inc., New York, N.Y.

Acknowledgments of Assistance

A great many people have helped me with this work. I wish I could express my gratitude to each of them in these pages, but it is obviously impractical. I have to be content with mentioning only a few.

The following generous souls from the academic field have helped me tremendously: Prof. Charles Workman, Chairman of the English Department, Samford University; Prof. K. L. Seshagiri Rao of the Department of Religion, University of Virginia; Prof. Jane Christian and Prof. John Hamer of the Department of Anthropology, University of Alabama at Birmingham (UAB); Prof. Jesse Milby of the Department of Psychiatry, UAB; and Prof. A. A. Khatri, Department of Sociology, UAB.

Prominent among my colleagues who lent their support in many ways are: Thomas Brecht, Ph.D., Michael Holt, Ph.D., Robert Durham, M. Div., Clarence McDanal, M.D., David Morrison, M.D., Mrs. Boots Groff, B.S.N., and Mrs. Irene Hamer, M.S.W.

I owe a great deal to several people from the field of religion: Rev. John Groff, Rev. Joseph Marino, Rev. Frank Muscolino, and Mrs. Norsat Scott.

My wife Anne Xavier, M.D., and my office manager Ms. Faye Stanley provided inspiration and support throughout the project. Special appreciation is due Mrs. Irma Cruise for editorial help, Mrs. Valerie Brechue and Ms. Mary Gustin for typing and gathering information, and Mr. James Travis, my publisher, for his creative efforts in giving final shape to this book.

INDEX OF NAMES

INDEX OF SUBJECTS

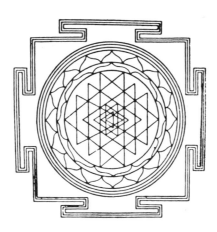